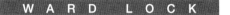

WARD LOCK

FAMILY HEALTH GUIDE

HEARING LOSS & TINNITUS

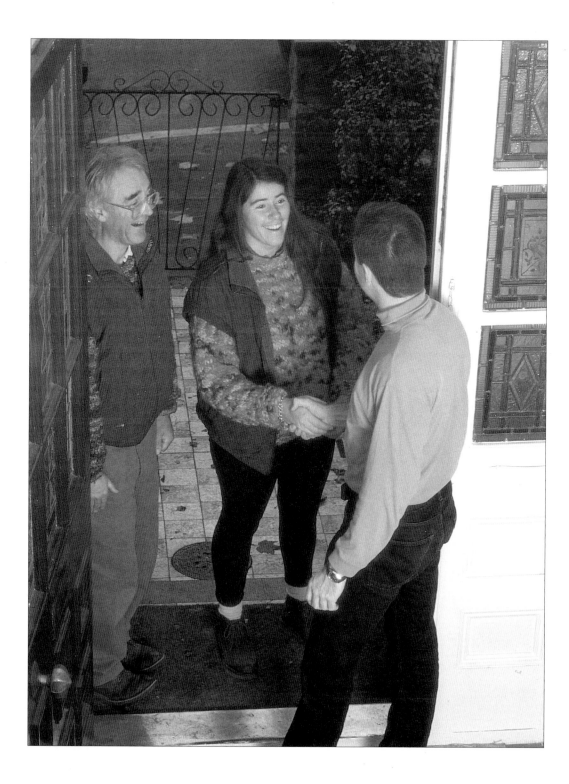

WARD LOCK

FAMILY HEALTH GUIDE

HEARING LOSS & TINNITUS

LORRAINE JEFFREY

IN ASSOCIATION WITH
THE ROYAL NATIONAL INSTITUTE
FOR DEAF PEOPLE

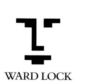

WARD LOCK

Lorraine Jeffrey

Lorraine Jeffrey is a hearing therapist who has worked for 12 years as part of a multi-disciplinary audiological rehabilitation team at the Royal National Throat, Nose and Ear Hospital, London. She also worked for the Royal National Institute for Deaf People for two years as an information development officer. She lives in London with her partner and two children.

A WARD LOCK BOOK

First published in the UK 1995
by Ward Lock
Wellington House
125 Strand
LONDON
WC2R 0BB

A Cassell Imprint

Distributed in the United States
by Sterling Publishing Co., Inc.
387 Park Avenue South, New York, NY 10016–8810

Distributed in Australia
by Capricorn Link (Australia) Pty Ltd
2/13 Carrington Road, Castle Hill NSW 2154

A British Library Cataloguing in Publication Data block for this book may be obtained from the British Library

ISBN 0 7063 7396 0
Designed by Lindsey Johns and typeset by The Design Revolution, Brighton
Printed and bound in Spain

Acknowledgements

The author would like to thank the Royal National Throat, Nose and Ear Hospital audiological rehabilitation team for their invaluable advice; and her family and friends for their unflagging support. Thanks are also due to the staff at the Institute of Laryngology photographic unit for the photographs reproduced on pages 10, 13, 22, 23, 26, 27, 30, 31, 33, 34, 35, 36, 37, 41, 55, 56, 74; and to Life File for supplying photographs reproduced on the following pages: 11, 59, 61, 67 (Nicola Sutton); 2, 20, 51 (Tim Fisher); 39 (Dave Thompson); 44 (Ray Ward); 46 (Mark Hibbert); 48 (S.L.P.S.); 63 (Richard Powers). Cover photograph: The Image Bank.

Contents

Introduction

You are reading this book because you have a reason to be interested in hearing loss and tinnitus. Your reason could be one of many. Perhaps you are thinking of a career working with people who have a hearing loss, but as yet you know nothing at all about the subject. You may have a relative or friend who is struggling with a newly acquired hearing aid and would very much like to learn what you can do to help them make the most of it. Or you may be worried that you yourself are developing a hearing loss but are unsure what to do about it – will a hearing aid help or not, and, more to the point, what is available? This book will help because it provides basic blocks of information on hearing aids and assistive listening devices and on how to develop effective communication strategies, as well as offering advice on ways of coping with tinnitus: a foundation of information which can be built upon.

Lorraine Jeffrey

Chapter one

The ear and how it works

Your ears are amazing features that allow you to enjoy a piano recital or join in a conversation as well as being aware of, say, birdsong or the approach of an ambulance. Of your five senses – sight, hearing, touch, smell and taste – hearing is perhaps the one most responsible for keeping you in touch with other people and the world around you. Your hearing enables you both to communicate and to have an awareness of the surrounding environment. This remarkable feat is achieved out of sight and very often out of mind; if your ears are working as they should, you do not have to make any effort at all to hear. Your ears are constantly flooded with the sounds present in your immediate environment, but you will not necessarily be conscious of hearing them. It is only when you listen or attend to a sound that you may actually become aware that you are using your sense of hearing.

The ear is an incredibly complex system which almost defies attempts to describe its structure without mention of how each particular part functions. However, in order to explain clearly the way in which the ear works, an attempt has been made to do precisely that: separate structure from function. Fortunately nature and to an extent medical convention allow the ear to be divided into three distinct sections, namely the outer, middle and inner ear. The structure of each section will be looked at in turn, and then the way in which each section functions will be explained.

It is important to note that in order for you to hear normally the structure of your ear must be intact and the function unimpaired.

Structure of the ear

The outer ear

The outer ear consists of the external ear (pinna) and the ear canal (external auditory meatus). The ear canal ends at the eardrum (tympanic membrane), which is the boundary between the outer and middle ear. The pinna, which is formed of springy cartilage covered in skin, has a unique complex shape, just like a fingerprint – no two ears are exactly alike. We are aware of sensations arising from the outer ear because the area is well supplied with nerves: anyone who has ever suffered from earache will readily agree that this is the case. The only muscles associated with the outer ear

The ear and how it works

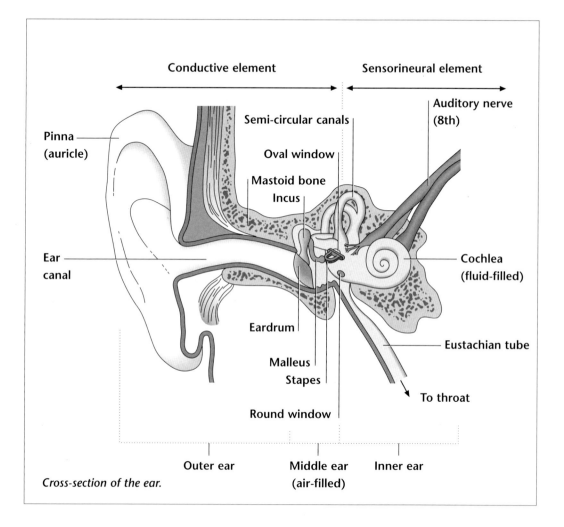

Cross-section of the ear.

are to be found just behind the pinna and these attach the ear to the skull. However, unlike in other mammals, such as dogs or cats, they do not perform any particular function except perhaps to allow people who can move them and hence wiggle their ears to amuse those who cannot!

The ear canal is approximately 2.5 cm/1 in in length. The outer third is, like the pinna, formed of cartilage and the inner portion is bony. The canal is lined with skin, the outer third of which bears a large number of fine hairs as well as two types of glands; one of these produces oil, the other wax or cerumen. It is interesting to note that the skin which lines the ear canal and covers the eardrum behaves slightly differently from skin elsewhere on the body. Normally as skin grows the dead cells are shed at the surface, but this would obviously create a serious problem in the restricted space of the ear canal. Instead of simply flaking off, therefore, dead skin migrates from the inner portion of the canal outwards, and this ensures that the canal does not become blocked during the natural process of skin growth.

The middle ear

The middle ear is the air-filled space, or tympanic cavity, situated behind the eardrum. It contains the three bones which make up the ossicular chain, muscles and nerves. The cavity is lined with a membrane which secretes mucus and the walls have a number of important features. These are the eustachian tube, which connects the middle ear to the back of the nose and throat, a small opening leading to the air-filled cells of the mastoid bone and two membrane-covered openings, called the oval and round windows. The chain of three bones connects the eardrum to the inner ear. The bone known as the malleus (or hammer) is attached by its handle to the eardrum, the incus (or anvil) is the second bone and the stapes (or stirrup) completes the chain with its footplate attached to the oval window of the inner ear. The ossicular chain is suspended in the cavity by ligaments and two small muscles maintain its rigidity.

Finally two main nerves run through the middle ear, one responsible for controlling facial expression and the other for relaying the sense of taste to the brain.

The inner ear

The inner ear is in fact one fluid-filled structure which has two sections: the cochlea (the organ of hearing) and the semi-circular canals (the organ of balance). The inner ear is separated from the middle ear by the oval and round windows, both covered by membranes which prevent the fluid from leaking out of the cochlea and semi-circular canals into the air-filled middle ear.

The cochlea is a coiled structure divided into two chambers containing a series of special membranes that are bathed in the fluid. The two chambers are separated by a ridge known as the organ of Corti; from this ridge protrude two types of cells called the inner hair cells and outer hair cells. These are your auditory sensory cells, whose function it is to send signals to the auditory nerve, commonly referred to as the eighth nerve. A normal cochlea contains approximately 3,000 inner hair cells and 12,000 outer hair cells, though a decline in numbers does occur as a natural consequence of the passage of time. It is inevitable and completely normal not to have as many hair cells at 50 years old as you did at 18, but it is reassuring to note that this depletion does not automatically result in a noticeable loss of hearing.

You rely for your sense of balance on the three semi-circular canals (mentioned again in Chapter two in connection with Menière's disease) and two additional bulbous structures called the saccule and utricle which are responsible for recording the motion and position of your head. The latter information is relayed to your brain by the vestibular branch of the auditory nerve.

The ear and how it works

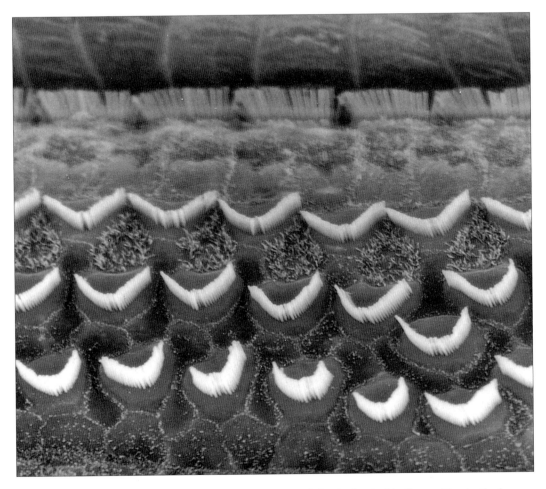

Rows of healthy inner and outer hair cells in the organ of Corti, situated in the cochlea in the inner ear. These are the sensory cells that change sounds into signals which are relayed to the brain.

How the ear works

The functions of the three sections of the ear can be divided conveniently into two elements: the conductive element (outer and middle ear) and the sensorineural element (inner ear). The conductive element is so called because the purpose of the outer and middle ear is to conduct external sounds to the inner ear. Once the sounds reach the inner ear, the cochlea,

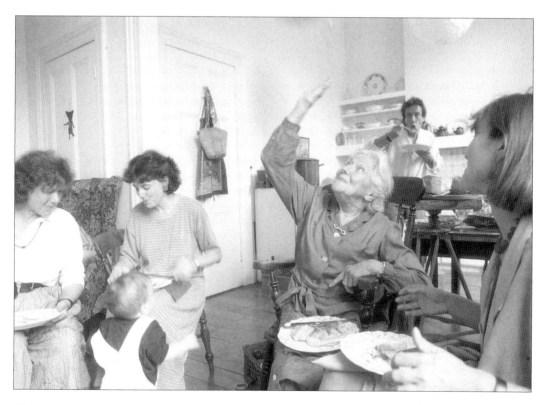

The depletion of hair cells that occurs naturally with age does not automatically result in a noticeable loss of hearing.

with its sensory cells (hair cells), changes the sounds into signals which can be relayed to your brain for processing via the auditory nerve: this is the sensorineural element of the sense of hearing.

Incidentally these terms are also used to describe types of hearing loss. If the outer or middle ear fails to function normally, any deficit of hearing arising from this malfunction is called a conductive loss. Similarly a hearing loss which is the consequence of a malfunction of the inner ear may be referred to as a

sensorineural loss of hearing (sometimes known as a nerve deafness). Chapter two covers types of hearing loss in more detail.

The conductive element

Outer ear

The pinna, with its shell-like convolutions, acts as a receptor for sounds. It is even believed that perhaps the shape of the human ear directs sound into the ear canal, a theory which may be supported by the existence of the oldest hearing aid in the world – a hand cupped

11

The ear and how it works

around the ear! This simple action produces a noticeable increase in sound level. The fact that you have two ears is of importance too, because both must work in order for you to determine where a sound comes from.

Sounds then travel down the ear canal to meet the eardrum, which absorbs them and responds by moving back and forth. To do so the eardrum must be intact and flexible. In order for sounds to reach the eardrum the ear canal must be free from obstructions and the eardrum must have air on both sides of it before it can move freely in response to the sounds meeting it.

In this connection mention should be made of ear wax. As already stated, wax production is a completely normal function of the ear canal. We all make wax, though the amount produced depends upon many factors and consequently can vary enormously. It protects the canal in a number of ways by collecting any debris which might enter the ears, plus the dead skin migrating out of the inner two-thirds. The wax is both anti-bacterial and anti-fungal as well as water-resistant. Suprisingly the presence of wax in the ear canal has no effect whatsoever on the hearing provided it does not completely block the canal.

The ear canal will become blocked with wax only if the natural process of migration and wax production is interrupted. It is completely unnecessary to attempt to clean your ear canals by inserting anything such as cotton-tipped buds: this simply results in wax being pushed back down the canals, and it can then become hard and impacted, perhaps eventually blocking the canals or causing discomfort because it is pressing on the eardrums. If you suspect that your ears are blocked with wax, it is always advisable to consult your family doctor before attempting any sort of home remedy. There is value in the old adage 'never put anything smaller than your elbow in your ear' – unless, of course, you are told otherwise by your doctor or audiologist.

Middle ear

The function of the middle ear is to transmit sounds and convert them into signals which are suitable for passage through the cochlea. Movement of the eardrum in response to sound produces a corresponding vibration of the bones in the ossicular chain, which in turn causes movement of the membrane of the oval window. The chain of bones must be intact and the middle ear cavity full of air in order for sounds to be transmitted effectively to the fluid of the inner ear. Air enters the cavity via the eustachian tube which opens and closes when you yawn or swallow: this ensures that the pressure inside the middle ear is more or less the same as that in the ear canal.

The sensorineural element

Inner ear

The movement of the membrane of the oval window causes the fluid in the cochlea to move against the hair cells, making them produce signals. These signals travel along the auditory nerve and are relayed to the brain to be processed and interpreted as sound. It is essential that the cochlea is healthy and that the signals produced by the hair cells reach the part of the brain responsible for hearing.

How hearing is measured

If your ears are working normally, you are able to hear an enormous range of sounds from the quiet buzz of a fly to thunder crashing during a storm. These and other sounds, such as the human voice, a dog barking or the noise of your car engine, reach your ears in the form of a wave of pressure travelling through the air.

They are complex sounds because they consist of combinations of the simplest elements of sound: puretones. It is your ears' ability to hear puretones, that very basic property of your hearing, which is used to determine the level or threshold of your hearing when you have a hearing test or audiogram. The puretone

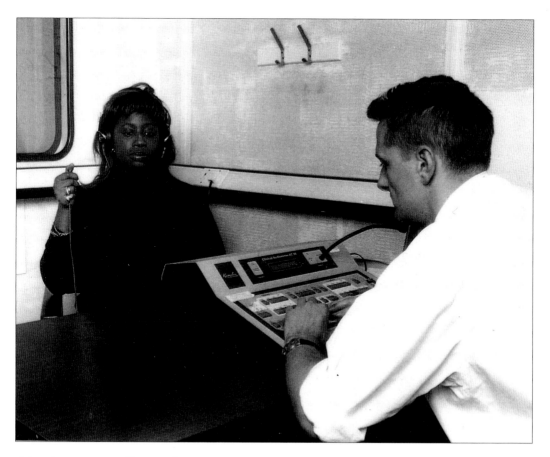

A hearing test, or audiogram, in progress.

The ear and how it works

audiogram (PTA) illustrated below shows the results of normal hearing. The symbols O and X simply indicate the response of the right and left ear respectively.

A puretone sound has two important variables: frequency (pitch) and amplitude (loudness). These are shown in the diagram below.

The pitch of a puretone is measured in hertz (Hz). A normal human ear can respond to a range of puretones from a very low tone (20Hz) to a very high tone (20,000Hz), but for the purposes of a hearing test a limited range of frequencies (tones) is used. The range tested is limited to those that are relevant to hearing human speech, so the puretone audiogram, a test routinely used in most clinics or hospitals internationally, covers only 125Hz to 8,000Hz.

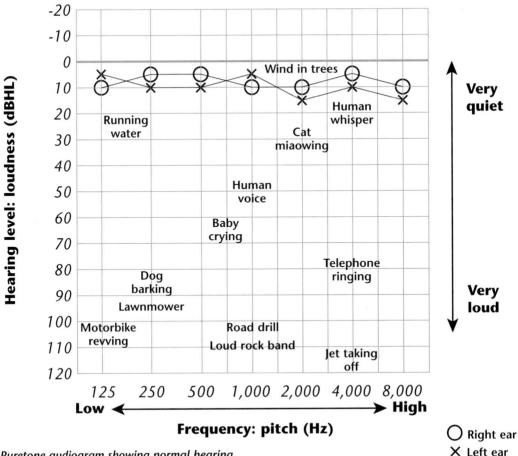

Puretone audiogram showing normal hearing.

○ Right ear
X Left ear

In fact your hearing may not be tested over all these frequencies, even though they are shown on the audiogram, because test protocols may differ from clinic to clinic, but essentially the audiologist aims to establish your level of hearing across a range of tones.

For the purposes of a hearing test the loudness of a puretone is measured using a scale which is relevant to the human ear, namely decibel hearing level (dBHL). The audiometer used to test your hearing is capable of producing puretone sounds from 0dBHL (quietest) to 120dBHL (extremely loud). The audiologist will be able to establish the level or threshold of your hearing accurately with your co-operation by noting your response to sounds which get progressively quieter.

Many people worry that the test results do not accurately represent their hearing, particularly if they also have tinnitus (ringing or whistling in the ear), because the test requires you to respond to the quietest sound that you can hear in order to establish your threshold of hearing and it is difficult to know sometimes whether you have actually heard a sound or not. However, this need not be a cause for concern as the audiologist uses a test procedure which shows very clearly when you can hear a sound and when you cannot. More information about hearing tests that the doctor may request as part of your consultation can be found in the following chapter.

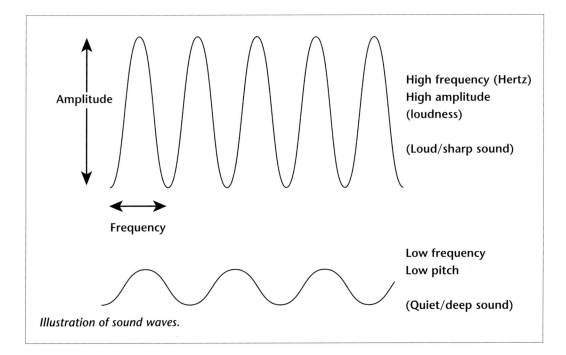

High frequency (Hertz)
High amplitude
(loudness)

(Loud/sharp sound)

Low frequency
Low pitch

(Quiet/deep sound)

Illustration of sound waves.

Chapter two
Hearing loss

As the preceding chapter showed, your ears are very complex and in order for you to hear normally they must work perfectly. But throughout your life your ears, in common with the rest of your body, are vulnerable to the effects of genetics, the environment, illness, accident and the relentless passage of time. It is not suprising therefore that, as a result of these influences acting either separately or together, you can develop a hearing loss at any time

Hearing level: loudness (dBHL)		
-20		
-10		
0		Normal
10		
20		
30	5.0 million	Mild
40		
50	2.2 million	
60		Moderate
70		
80	240,000	Severe
90		
100		
110	60,000	Profound
120		

125   250   500   1,000 2,000 4,000 8,000
Frequency: pitch (Hz)

Categories of hearing loss.   *Source:* British Society of Audiology

from the beginning to the end of your life. In fact it has been estimated that up to 40 per cent of adults over the age of 65 years and approximately 7.5 million of the total adult population in Great Britain have some degree of hearing loss.

What sort of hearing loss do I have?

It will become clear during the course of this chapter that it is possible to categorize hearing loss in a number of ways. So in order to avoid confusion, terms that you may encounter in this book and any subsequent reading, or during consultations, are set out below for your information. A hearing loss may be defined as follows:

● according to which part of the auditory system has been affected – if the structure of your outer or middle ear is disrupted, the loss is conductive; if your cochlea fails to function normally, the loss is sensorineural;

● according to when the loss developed – if you are born with or develop a loss very shortly after birth this is called a congenital loss; if it develops at any point later on, it is called an acquired loss; and acquired loss may be further defined by the time when it was acquired – before the development of language, it is known as a pre-lingual loss; if after language development, as post-lingual loss;

● according to the degree of the hearing loss – it may be classified as mild, moderate, severe or profound;

● according to whether the loss affects one ear (known as unilateral loss) or both ears (known as bilateral loss).

The causes of hearing loss

What can cause a hearing loss? The answer is anything that interferes at all with the way your ears work. The potential causes are so numerous that it would be impossible to include every conceivable one within the confines of this chapter: the tables are by no means exhaustive and it must be stressed that the treatments outlined are only possibilities. It is essential that the diagnosis of the cause of a hearing loss and any subsequent medical treatment of the problem are carried out by a suitably qualified doctor.

Conductive hearing loss

Many of the causes of conductive hearing loss are amenable to medical treatment, often with a very successful outcome. However, it is important to note that this type of loss is by its very nature easily remedied by use of a hearing aid. The ear's failure to conduct the sound to the inner ear can in some cases be overcome by simply making the sounds louder. Hearing aids and how to make the most of them are covered in some detail in the next two chapters.

Hearing loss

Causes and treatment of conductive hearing loss

Cause	Treatment
Obstruction of the ear canal by wax, water, foreign object	Syringing, suction or manual removal under microscope
Inflammation of the skin of the ear canal causing an irritation and/or swelling (otitis externa)	Prescription of medication aiming to reduce the symptoms
Perforation of the eardrum as a result of trauma, e. g. sudden change of pressure or infection	Prescription of medication or, if persistent, surgical treatment to repair the drum (tympanoplasty)
Infection of the middle ear – common in children, often in association with a cold or tonsillitis (acute otitis media)	Possible prescription of medication or allowing the infection to run its course
Chronic otitis media or glue ear (covered in more detail in Chapter six) due to allergy, infection or eustachian tube dysfunction	Possible prescription of medication, restricting exposure to potential allergens, surgical resolution by insertion of grommets
Persistent inflammation of the middle ear with unresolved perforation of the eardrum (chronic suppurative otitis media)	Precription of medication and/or surgical repair of the drum
Infection or failure of eustachian tube function (eustachian tube dysfunction)	Medication for infection and/or instruction on inflation of the tube
Abnormal growth of bone, usually involving the third bone in the ossicular chain – the stapes, or stirrup (otosclerosis)	Possible surgical intervention (stapedectomy) or provision of a hearing aid
Ossicular discontinuity, possibly congenital or the result of trauma such as a blow to the ear	Possible surgical repair (ossiculoplasty)
Congenital malformation of the outer and/or middle ear	Surgical reconstruction

Sensorineural hearing loss

The causes of sensorineural hearing loss are as numerous as the causes of conductive loss but unfortunately far less amenable to medical treatment. When the inner ear is damaged in any way, the result more often than not is permanent: it is simply not possible surgically to repair or replace hair cells that no longer function. So the table below lists mainly causes, mentioning treatment only occasionally. Yet a great deal can be done to minimize the impact of a hearing loss on your life. Chapter four offers practical advice on coping with, and getting the most from a hearing aid.

Causes and some treatment of sensorineural hearing loss

Cause	Treatment
Exposure to noise	
Viral/bacterial infection	
Congenital	
Hereditary factors, e.g. Paget's disease	
Ototoxic drugs (if you are concerned that any medication you are taking is affecting your hearing consult your family doctor)	
Menière's disease – fluctuating hearing loss associated with attacks of dizziness	Possible palliative treatment of symptoms
Acoustic neuroma – rare benign tumour of the acoustic nerve	Possible surgical removal
Head injury	
Vascular incident	
Surgical trauma	
Perilymph leak – a leak of the fluid contained in the cochlea from the oval window	Possible prescription of medication or surgical treatment

Hearing loss

How do I know if I have a loss?

A hearing loss may develop very suddenly or obviously, accompanied perhaps by a heavy cold or some form of discomfort such as a sensation of blockage, pain or discharge, noises in the ears, or unsteadiness. Most people experiencing any of these symptoms would seek the opinion of their family doctor, whose treatment may well resolve the problem. However, all too often the signs indicating the existence of a hearing loss are not so obvious. It is after all extremely easy to blame difficulty hearing, say, the dialogue of a television play on the actors' poor diction or the excessively loud background music. In fact unless someone tells you that you did not hear the doorbell or asks why you did not answer the phone you may remain unaware that there is a problem – you cannot know that you missed a sound you did not hear! It is the nature of hearing loss to be gradual and insidious, and this is particularly true of a sensorineural loss which rarely manifests itself with a fanfare.

Some signs that may indicate a hearing loss

Do you:
- need the television sound volume higher than is comfortable for others?
- request frequent repetition or sometimes misunderstand people?

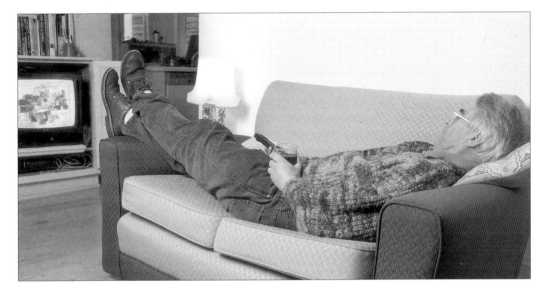

One sign of hearing loss is needing to turn up the television sound so that it is uncomfortable for others.

• find that people complain about unanswered telephones and doorbells?

• avoid social occasions or noisy situations?

• wish that others would stop mumbling when they speak?

• find following a group conversation difficult?

• find it difficult to determine where a sound came from?

• worry that your memory or concentration is failing?

If the answer to any of these questions is yes, it is possible that you have developed a hearing loss. It is important to seek advice as soon as possible, because ignoring any of the difficulties mentioned will not improve matters. Research has shown that it may take a person as long as 15 years from the onset of experiencing hearing difficulties to decide to try to deal with them. Unfortunately the passage of time tends only to compound the problems that can arise as a result of hearing loss.

The factors that can contribute to this reluctance are complex and most of them are completely understandable. Perhaps you are worried about exposing yourself to the social stigma associated with deafness, which sadly still prevails despite campaigns and education. This book aims to provide you with an arsenal to counter other people's ignorance of the needs of the deaf and hearing impaired, as well as to help you develop strategies for coping with your loss. You may object to a hearing aid on aesthetic grounds. Unlike spectacles, hearing aids have yet to achieve fashion accessory status; they are, however, getting smaller. It may be helpful to bear in mind that other people are more likely to notice that you are unable to hear properly than they are to notice your hearing aid. Solutions to the problems do exist and are never as daunting as anticipated.

Possible consequences of not dealing with a hearing loss

• Relatives and friends may become irritated and intolerant.

• Increased social isolation (doorbells, telephones unanswered).

• Annoyance of family and neighbours (television sound too high).

• Reduction of activities (cinema, theatre, classes).

• Difficulties at work resulting from misunderstandings or mistakes.

• Exposure to danger through reduced awareness of warning sounds.

• Difficulties adapting to amplified sound.

• Development of feelings of frustration, anger or anxiety.

Hearing loss

Seeing the family doctor

If you suspect that you are developing a hearing loss or are told by those closest to you that you appear to be experiencing difficulty hearing, the first step should be to see your family doctor. He or she will be able to examine your ears and provide treatment if appropriate – perhaps the removal of impacted wax or the prescription of antibiotics for an active infection. If the cause of your loss is not amenable to treatment, he or she will be able to arrange a referral to an appropriate specialist for an opinion should you desire one.

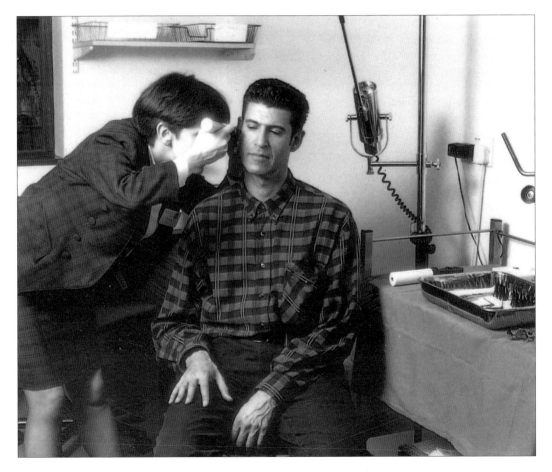

A doctor examining a patient with hearing problems.

Seeing a specialist

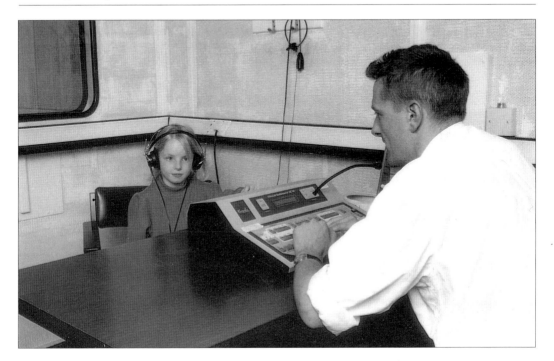

An audiologist testing a child's hearing.

Your referral will usually be to a doctor specializing in disorders of the ear, nose and throat (the medical term used to refer to this field of medicine is otorhinolaryngology). The specialist may be any one of the following:

● an otolaryngologist (often an ENT surgeon);
● a neuro-otologist (a doctor specializing in disorders of the ear and balance);
● an audiological physician (usually a doctor with a particular interest in audiological/aural rehabilitation).

Other professionals you might encounter include:

● an audiologist – responsible for diagnostic tests, assessment for and provision of hearing aids (in some countries he or she may be involved in rehabilitation programmes);
● a hearing therapist – provides pre-fitting and supportive counselling, programmes of rehabilitation, optimization and fitting of hearing aids, assessment for provision of assistive devices;
● a speech and language therapist (may be called speech, language and hearing therapist in some countries and be involved in provision of hearing aids and rehabilitation) – responsible

Hearing loss

for providing speech therapy.

Also noteworthy is the fact that you may not see the specialist but a member of his or her team of doctors. The majority of hospitals and clinics have a policy that staff members wear identity badges, but if you are unsure about the identity or role of the person dealing with you it is always worth enquiring.

The consultation

The aim of the doctor faced with your complaint of difficulty in hearing will be to establish the following facts:
● the level of your hearing loss;
● whether it is conductive or sensorineural;
● the cause of the loss (if possible – it cannot always be discovered);
● whether the loss is causing any problems.

To do so the doctor will examine your ears using an otoscope, take a medical history and request hearing tests such as a puretone audiogram (PTA) and tympanometry (see the section below on hearing tests). Any subsequent treatment will depend upon the results of these investigations and could involve medical treatment or more tests. But what if the outcome of your consultation is that further medical intervention is neither required nor appropriate because you have been diagnosed as having a hearing loss that is not amenable to treatment by the doctor? You may well be disappointed that nothing can be done medically to resolve your problem, perhaps somewhat stunned by the suggestion that a hearing aid might help and wondering where you go from here and whether any other help is available.

What happens next?

To a large extent that depends upon the answers to a number of questions, most of which centre on what you want and need as well, of course, as on the resources available. The questions might include the following:
● Is a hearing aid is appropriate for you?
● Do you want a hearing aid?
● What sort of difficulties are you experiencing as a result of your hearing loss?
● How do you feel about your hearing loss?
● Do you and/or your family members need to talk about ways to cope with communication difficulties?
● Would you like to talk to someone about hearing aids before trying one?
● Is the doctor willing and able to refer you on to an appropriate professional such as an audiologist or hearing therapist for a trial of a hearing aid and advice on coping with a hearing loss?

In an ideal world you would be able to spend time with the doctor discussing your options before answering any of those questions, followed by pre-fitting counselling, supported trial of an appropriate hearing aid, and advice on assistive devices (such as for television viewing) and how to obtain them. As we do not live in an ideal world and a common experience for hearing aid users is to be very disappointed with their aid, the next two chapters aim to remedy the shortfall.

Hearing tests

Hearing tests are carried out by an audiologist, usually in soundproof conditions, and can be divided into two types.

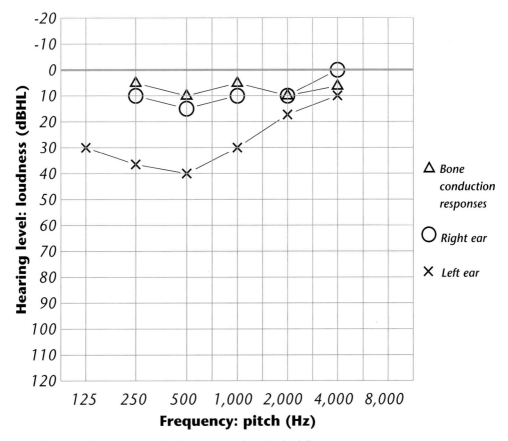

Puretone audiogram showing a conductive hearing loss in the left ear.

Subjective tests

These require you to wear headphones and respond to a signal by pressing a button. The audiologist will also place a small vibrating pad on the bone behind your ear to test how well you hear sounds via the bones of your skull. The results will show clearly whether you have a conductive or sensorineural loss. Examples of subjective tests are a puretone audiogram, Bekesy test and speech audiogram.

A speech audiogram provides useful information about your ability to discriminate speech sounds; this will normally be unaffected by a conductive loss. The test results will show a normal-shaped curve but displaced to the right, indicating that you simply need sounds louder. The curve that has rolled over clearly shows that no matter how loud a sound is made it is not heard clearly. This is typical of many sensorineural hearing losses, which result in a reduced ability to discriminate sounds. Chapter four offers advice on coping with this.

Hearing loss

Objective tests

These do not require you to respond actively to a signal but need your co-operation as they can involve painless procedures such as wearing electrodes or tolerating insertion of a small rubber probe into the ear canal. Examples of objective tests are evoked response audiometry, tympanometry and otoacoustic emissions.

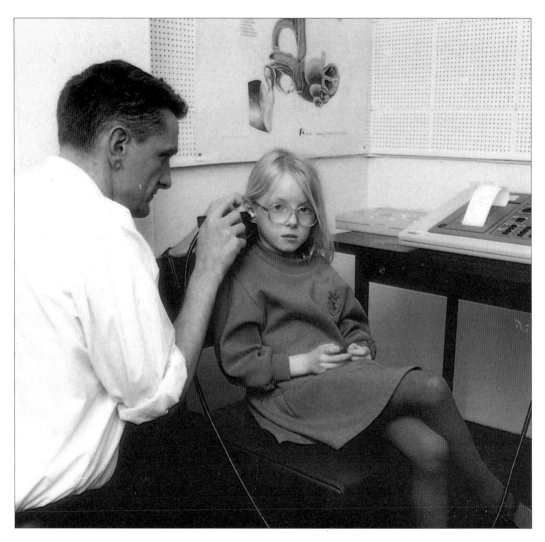

A child undergoing typanometry, a test of middle ear function.

Chapter three

Equipment

Daily life is full of situations that are undoubtedly more difficult to cope with if you have a hearing loss. These can range from hearing the alarm clock in the morning to conversations, or from using the telephone to watching television. Can anything be done to help you overcome these difficulties?

The answer is: a great deal. An amazing array of equipment, designed to help you cope with your hearing loss, is available, all of which could be described as aids to hearing. However, the term hearing aid is usually reserved only for the devices that can be worn by you as you go about your daily life. Reflecting this, the first

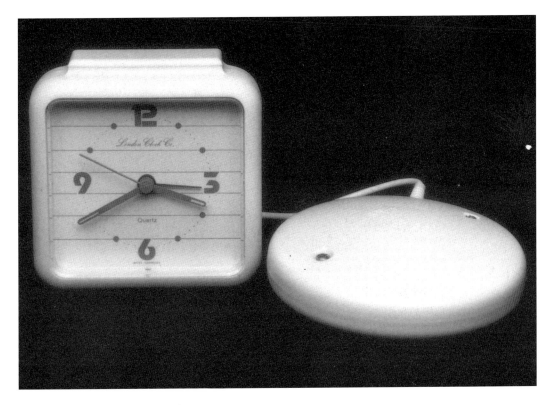

Alarm clock with vibrating pad.

Equipment

section of this chapter, called simply 'Hearing aids', describes the range of devices that have been designed principally to aid communication. The second section, entitled 'Assistive listening devices', covers equipment that has been developed to ease daily living.

You may well be wondering why you might need anything other than your hearing aid, and it is possible that your hearing aid will satisfy all your needs. In fact a hearing aid is sometimes simply not enough to solve the problem completely: for instance, wearing an aid at night so that you do not miss the alarm in the morning is likely to be extremely uncomfortable. In addition a hearing aid may not be suitable or desired, but certain activities still present particular problems, such as hearing on the telephone or watching television. Many arguments can erupt over something as small as the volume button on the remote control or the constant ringing of an unanswered telephone!

Hearing aids

The range of hearing aids available today is so vast that it is probably safe to state that the majority of people with a hearing loss, whether it is conductive or sensorineural, could benefit from using an appropriate, properly fitted aid. Making the decision to try a hearing aid is never easy and will probably involve a great deal of wrestling with your thoughts and feelings. If you have made that decision, you are more than half-way to using a hearing aid successfully, because the first hurdle is motivation. It is virtually impossible to force anyone to use a hearing aid – you have to want to wear one. The second hurdle is your expectations: it is impossible to overemphasize that these must be realistic.

However, an appropriate aid fitted and adjusted to suit your hearing loss and needs by a skilled audiologist or dispenser (if you are purchasing privately) can improve matters immeasurably. In time you will wonder how on earth you managed before and why you did not

What to expect from a hearing aid

- A hearing aid is simply an amplifier – admittedly very small and in some instances quite sophisticated, but nevertheless an amplifier.
- The aid can do only what its name suggests – aid the hearing you have left by making sounds louder.
- It is still not possible, as yet, to tailor amplified sound to replace your lost hearing exactly.
- It can take time, sometimes months, to adjust to amplified sound. This is particularly true in the case of a long-standing hearing loss.

try one sooner! It probably won't be perfect, but you will find that conversations are once again pleasurable and some of the problems you have been experiencing will fade away. Chapter four offers ideas on how to get the most out of your hearing aid and suggests solutions to some of the common problems that users can face.

Some notes on purchasing an aid privately

Deciding to purchase a hearing aid privately could be compared to entering a minefield, because a mistake can be very costly. Hearing aids are without doubt expensive in the UK, where prices can range from about £250 for a basic model to £1,200 for a top-of-the-range device such as a programmable aid with a remote control. When you are considering purchasing anything, you can usually shop around before making your decision. You also know what to expect from your purchase when you get it home: if you buy, say, a washing machine and it fails to get the clothes clean or leaks all over the floor, you know that it is not doing its job. Purchasing a hearing aid can be a little more difficult. Shopping around is not so easy and if you have never worn a hearing aid before how will you know if it is doing its job properly? Can you be sure that the aid is the most suitable one for you?

It is important to know the golden rules before embarking on the purchase of a hearing aid, not least because it can take time to learn the answers to these two questions, but also because hearing aid manufacturers produce very convincing advertisements proclaiming the benefits to be gained from their particular product and the people who sell the aids can be very persuasive.

The golden rules

1 Find a reputable dispenser This is not always easy, but word of mouth is a start – do you have a friend who is happy with their dispenser? If not, choosing a dispenser who has a base (perhaps a shop or practice) is a good policy: if you know where they are, you can go back to them if you have a problem!

2 Check the dispenser's credentials Regulatory bodies exist in most countries. In the UK, for example, a properly qualified dispenser should be registered with the Hearing Aid Council (address on page 78).

3 Do not sign anything before you read the small print. This may seem obvious, but many people do and find that they are stuck with an aid with which they are very unhappy.

4 Take someone along A family member or friend may counter any high-pressure sales tactics – it is easy to be swayed when you are unsure.

5 Insist on a trial period This should be a minimum of 30 days with a guaranteed refund of any deposit: adjusting to wearing an aid and hearing amplified sound does take time.

6 Insist on an after-sales service This is essential because your aid may need adjustment, hearing aids require maintenance, ear moulds do not last forever and you will definitely need to replace batteries!

If you stick to these rules, your experience of puchasing and using your aid should be a happy and successful one.

Equipment

Types of hearing aid

Hearing aids can be grouped into those worn on the head and those worn on the body. They vary in size from the completely invisible when worn, such as the deep canal aid which is tiny, to modern-day body-worn devices that are the size of a credit card in area but rather thicker. They can also vary in colour, in the amount of amplification provided and in the number of additional controls and facilities offered.

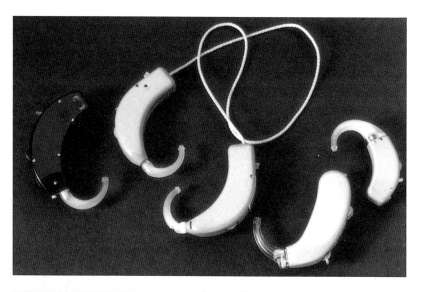

A range of behind-the-ear (BTE) hearing aids.

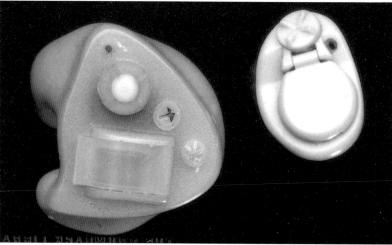

An in-the-ear (ITE) hearing aid (left) and an in-the-canal (ITC) hearing aid.

Head-worn or ear-level hearing aids

As their names suggest these hearing aids are worn on, in or near your ear. The photographs on page 30 show some of the different types available. They can range from those worn behind the ear (BTE), sometimes called postaural (a well-fitting ear mould is a crucial element of a postaural system: without it amplified sound would not reach its destination, your inner ear), to those worn in the ear (ITE) and in the canal (ITC). A BTE can be standard- or mini-sized – that shown in the photograph on the right is of a standard size attached to a shell ear mould. Although a mould is not required for an ITE or ITC, an impression of your ear is.

In some countries, most notably the USA and Australia, the majority of aids fitted are either ITE or ITC, but it should be noted that this type of aid will not suit everyone. This is because their small size limits the number and size of components that can be incorporated, which restricts the amount of amplified sound these hearing aids can provide. The aids are normally suitable only for mild to moderate hearing loss and it may not be possible to have a 'T' switch or an on/off switch – opening the battery compartment may be the only way to turn the aid off! Also handling a very small hearing aid demands a reasonable degree of manual dexterity.

An additional group of aids that can be called head-worn are the spectacle aids – in effect BTE aids attached to the arms of spectacles. Head-band bone-conduction devices are most suitable for people who have a conductive hearing loss and are unable to benefit from amplification via ear-worn aids. With these, sounds reach the inner ear via the bone of the skull (by bone conduction) rather than along the ear canal (by air conduction).

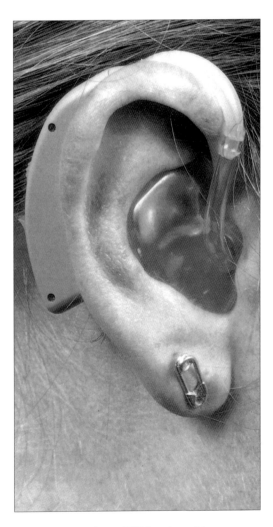

A woman wearing a BTE hearing aid.

Equipment

The ear mould

All the aids mentioned so far, with the exception of bone-conduction devices, require that an impression of your ear is taken. For ITEs and ITCs this will ensure that the casing fits your ear exactly. For BTE hearing aids an ear mould is crucial to successful use of the aid because it is the mould that carries the amplified sound to your ear and ensures that the aid stays put. It is essential that your ear mould fits well and is inserted correctly for two reasons:

- **Your physical comfort** – a badly fitting mould or one that is not in your ear properly will cause discomfort.
- **Quality of sound** – if the mould does not fit your ear exactly, amplified sound will not reach its destination (your eardrum in the first instance). This means that sound leaks back out of your ear, often causing the dreaded feedback, a high-pitched whistling noise.

Modifications

Modifying the ear mould can increase physical comfort and improve sound quality. For example, a vent or additional hole through the mould can relieve the sensation of blockage experienced by some hearing aid users. A larger vent can have the effect of reducing the impact of low-frequency sounds, whereas shaping or horning the end of the mould can have the effect of enhancing high-frequency sounds. It is important to let your audiologist or dispenser know if you are unhappy with your aid for any reason because there may be a solution to the problem – it could be as simple as replacing your mould with a new one.

The impression

Having an impression taken for the first time can be quite a bizarre experience. After all, it is not every day that you allow someone to fill your ear with something akin to a child's modelling clay! Your ear canal will be examined to ensure that it is free from wax before a small foam plug attached to a thread is inserted into the canal. It may feel as though this is being pushed down on to your eardrum, but in fact the audiologist pushes it in only as far as necessary to obtain a good impression. A soft material is then syringed into your canal and most of the pinna and left for a few minutes to firm up before being removed. The result will be a type of negative of your ear which will be sent to an ear-mould laboratory to be made up or, in the case of an ITE, to the hearing aid manufacturer.

Special features

At its most basic a hearing aid will consist of a microphone, an amplifier, a receiver and a power source, but advances in technology have meant that it is possible to incorporate features allowing manipulation of the amplified sound. These features are sometimes referred to as preset controls because the audiologist/ dispenser adjusts or presets them for you in accordance with your needs when fitting your aid. Some can be used to alter the quantity of sound your aid produces and others the quality of that sound, for example:

- **Automatic gain control** This allows the aid to be set so that sounds are kept at a comfortable level automatically by compressing the sound wave without distortion. It is a

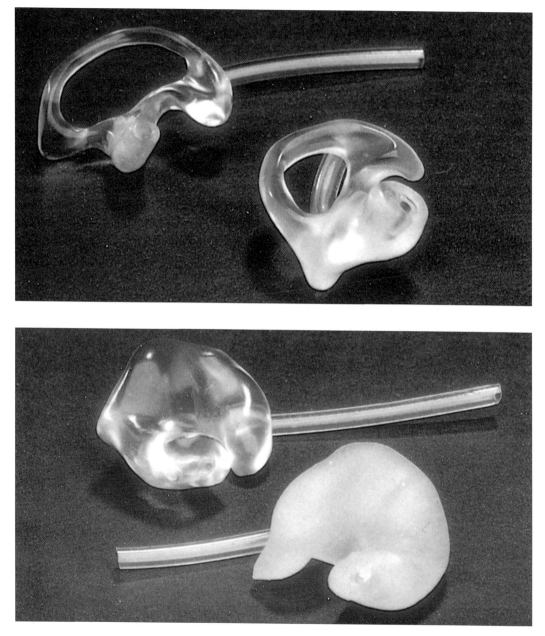

A range of ear moulds.

Equipment

useful feature to have if you are susceptible to loud noise causing discomfort.

● **Peak clipping** This is a similar type of feature but, as its name suggests, sound waves are clipped to prevent them becoming too loud. This can, however, sometimes cause distortion.

● **Tone controls** Used to alter the quality of the sounds by either reducing or increasing the amount of low or high frequencies produced.

● **Programmable aid** This type of hearing aid offers the wearer a choice of different presets. The dispenser can programme the hearing aid to suit different situations: for example, setting 1 will be most appropriate for television viewing but setting 2 best for conversation in background noise. These aids are often sold in conjunction with a remote control, a separate device that allows you to change between the different programmes. It is important to note that while these aids utilize digital technology, they are not actually digital hearing aids.

Body-worn hearing aids and communicators

A reasonable rule of thumb that can be applied to hearing aids is that the larger they are, the

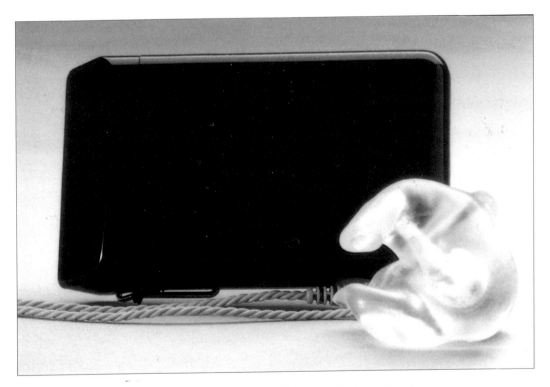

A body-worn hearing aid pictured with an ear mould to show their relative sizes.

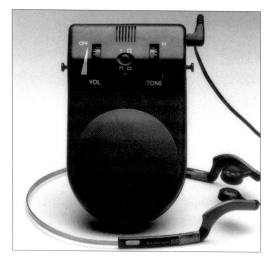

A communicator – a useful aid if other forms of amplification are unsuitable.

more powerful they are, so more often than not a body-worn hearing aid may be needed if you have a very profound loss. Nonetheless there are some extremely powerful postaural aids available. In some ways a body-worn aid is as discreet as an ITE, because only the mould and receiver need be visible. The need for powerful amplification may not be the only consideration: a body-worn aid may be more appropriate if the wearer has difficulty physically managing anything smaller.

Communicators are very basic hearing aids that can be used wearing headphones. This of course limits the amount of amplification they provide. Nevertheless communicators are very useful if using any other form of amplification is not possible.

Assistive listening devices

Are you worrying about or having difficulty hearing any of the following sounds with or without your hearing aid:
- Your alarm clock?
- The telephone ringing?
- The person speaking on the telephone?
- The smoke alarm at night?
- Your baby crying at night?
- People speaking during meetings at work?
- The cinema or theatre?
- The television or radio?
- The doorbell?

If the answer to any of these questions is yes, there are solutions to the problem. If you are unsure whether there are difficulties in your life as a result of hearing loss, consulting others can sometimes reveal as yet unrecognized problem areas.

One of the obvious solutions to the problem of not hearing something is to make it louder, so many assistive devices are designed to amplify. However, this may not be either possible or desirable: for example, in the case of a person with no useful hearing who wishes to use a telephone, an amplified handset would be redundant. The alternative is to change the signal from an auditory one to either a visual or physical one (that is, vibration). Many devices therefore utilize flashing lights or vibrating pads to alert you to the presence of a sound. The following list suggests different solutions for common problem areas.

Equipment

Alarms

You no longer need to worry about failing to hear your alarm clock or baby alarm if you have one that vibrates or flashes. Most fire alarms can be adapted to give a visual signal, and vibrating versions of smoke alarms are becoming increasingly available.

Doorbells

Missing the doorbell can be as frustrating for you as it is for the caller, so solve the problem with a louder bell or extensions in key rooms, or perhaps have a flashing-light system installed.

Telephone

The scourge of our modern society or an essential lifeline to family and friends? Whichever of these descriptions applies to the telephone, your hearing loss can make hearing it ring and using it difficult. Most telephone companies produce catalogues of their products which include louder-ringing phones, extension bells, and flashing-light systems – all designed to help you hear the phone ring. It is also possible to have a phone with an amplifier and coupler built into the handset or an additional ear piece for binaural use. For completely deaf people a textphone means contact with other textphone users and with conventional phones if a textphone relay system exists, such as Typetalk in Britain.

Television

For people whose hearing loss has reduced their viewing pleasure, an enormous number of listening devices is available ranging from a simple headphone system connecting the

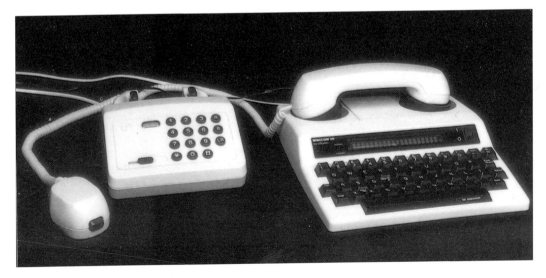

The Minicom, an example of a textphone.

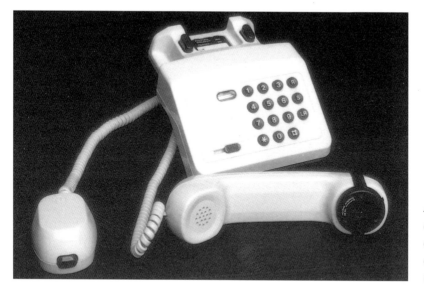

A telephone with an additional ear piece and a portable amplifier in place of the hand set.

viewer to the television, to infra-red systems that do not have cumbersome wires. If you use a hearing aid, a room loop may be a solution to your difficulty provided your aid has a 'T' switch.

Induction loop system

A loop system is a means of connecting a hearing aid user directly to a source of sound, provided their aid has a 'T' switch. Sound from any source – a television, a speaker at the cinema, even directly from a microphone – can be fed into the loop amplifier. This converts the sound signal into a current flowing through a wire, which can be any size small enough to go around your neck or large enough to go around an auditorium. The current in the wire sets up a magnetic field around the wire which the hearing aid on 'T' can pick up and convert back

into sound. The beauty of this system is that it enables the hearing aid user to hear sound directly from the source unaffected by distance from the sound and without interference from background noise.

This type of system has many applications and can often be found in cinemas and ticket sales booths (for example at rail stations). It can be used in meetings if connected into a microphone.

Communication support

Last but by no means least, the definition of assistance is extended to include help that can be provided by others in some situations where a device would be of no use. This help could be in the form of either a lipspeaker (a person who repeats very clearly and verbatim the words of another), sign language interpreter or notetaker.

Chapter four

Practical advice on coping with a hearing loss

Living with a hearing loss can be difficult whether it has crept up gradually, which is extremely common, or has arisen suddenly as a result of an illness or accident. This is because a fundamental part of our life has been affected – our ability to communicate. It is all too easy to take this ability for granted when we are not having any difficulty holding a conversation in a noisy place or using the telephone, and when we feel in touch with the world around us. But a hearing loss can affect our ability to communicate at many different levels with serious consequences, partly as a result of the fact that very few people know what to do when communication breaks down.

Communication necessarily involves another person, so you will not be the only one affected by the difficulties that can arise as a result of your hearing loss. Your family, friends and perhaps work colleagues will all have to adjust, and because communication is a two-way process they, like you, will need to learn to utilize tactics that can be used to improve day-to-day life. You are probably very aware that

your hearing aid has its limitations, because it does not always help as much as you would like in situations with high levels of background noise or in groups of people or where you are some distance from the speaker. Others, however, may not be aware of these limitations and consequently will expect too much of you and your aid when you are wearing it, so this chapter is as much for them as for you.

Many elements contribute to coping successfully with hearing loss. These include use of an aid, developing appropriate tactics to improve communication, provision of assistive devices (covered in Chapter three) and, last but not least, the support and understanding of others. When all these elements are combined, you will find that coping with your hearing loss is no longer quite so difficult. This chapter suggests strategies that will enable you to get the most from your hearing aid and tactics that you and others can use to improve communication in a variety of every-day situations.

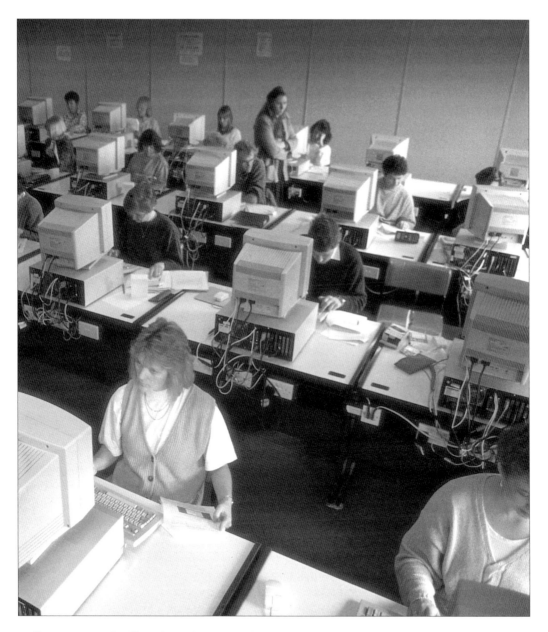

Colleagues at work will need to adjust to the fact that you have a hearing loss and adopt tactics to make communication as easy as possible.

Practical advice on coping with a hearing los

How to make the most of your hearing aid

It may seem an obvious statement, but in order to benefit from using a hearing aid you have to wear it! It is a sad fact that many people have a hearing aid which is kept in a box in a drawer, pocket or handbag only for occasions when they feel they really need it, such as that all-important family gathering, a crucial meeting at work or a long-awaited visit to the theatre. But they are often suprised and disappointed that the aid did not help as much as they expected: it was difficult to hear with everyone chatting, background noise in the office was overwhelming or the seats were too far away from the stage – so it's back to the drawer, pocket or handbag for the hearing aid. This sort of occasional use will inevitably result in lack of satisfaction with your hearing aid, because learning to use and to cope with amplified sound takes time and, as with learning any other skill, involves hard work. That is where the three Ps come into play: practice, patience and perseverance. Exercising them is vital if you are to use your aid successfully.

● **Practice** Using an aid requires practice. Wear it every day initially for one hour at a time, gradually increasing the length of time worn daily to the whole day if possible. Listening practice is also necessary, because amplified sound seems different at first, so you need to attempt using your aid initially in quiet indoor situations before subjecting yourself to background noise and the great outdoors. This will ensure that you gradually become accustomed to the background sounds of daily life and learn to keep them there – in the background! Make a mental list of the environmental sounds that you know you will be exposed to or need to hear in your home and workplace: for example, the doorbell, the telephone, water running, sounds of household or office/workshop appliances in use, traffic noise in the background and so on. Then ask yourself two questions regarding each sound:
1 What does it sound like when I'm wearing my aid?
2 Will I recognize the sound the next time I'm wearing my aid?
This exercise will ensure that you are not distacted by the extraneous sounds of every-day life such as the dishwasher pumping out while you are in mid-conversation with a friend in the kitchen.

● **Patience** Be patient with yourself. The process of adjustment does take time, and it can help if you explain this to others. Coping with a hearing loss is a gruelling business and can be tiring, so set your own pace.

● **Perseverence** Many people find using their aid difficult at first. You may, for instance, feel awkward handling it, feel that it is enormous and that everyone notices it. Rest assured they do not – looking at another person's ears is not the first thing people usually do when engaging in conversation. If you should notice someone staring at your ear, it is likely to be an audiologist or hearing therapist curious about the type of aid you have! Do not give up: you *will* become increasingly comfortable with your aid and more confident in your ability to use it effectively.

Dealing with problems

Common problems with hearing aids

- Whistling.

- Distortion of sound.

- Loud sounds may be painful.

- Lack of clarity.

- Poor sound quality.

- Background noise.

- Discomfort and irritation.

You know by now that the path to getting the most out of your aid is uphill and unfortunately one that is likely to be strewn with the odd boulder or two that will have to be negotiated. You will not necessarily encounter all of the problems listed in the box above and indeed may not have any at all. However, they are common, so you are not alone if you are struggling to find your way around any of them. The following section on potential causes and possible solutions should be useful whether you are having a particular difficulty or are a new hearing aid user who is not sure whether you are simply experiencing teething problems or should be complaining to your audiologist or dispenser.

Causes and solutions
Whistling

Whistling may be feedback resulting from amplified sound leaking from your ear back into the hearing aid when it is turned up to a particular volume. The most likely cause is an incorrectly fitted ear mould or ITE/ITC: either it has not been inserted properly or it no longer fits your ear well enough.

Another common cause of whistling can be

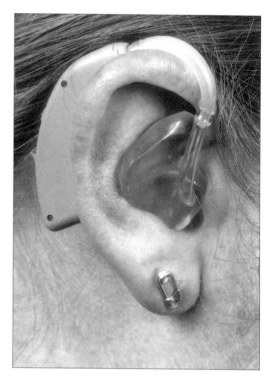

An incorrectly inserted ear mould can cause whistling.

Practical advice on coping with a hearing loss

a build-up of wax in your ear canal. Before rushing to your family doctor for an ear check or resorting to home remedies, however, try the following solutions:

1 Ensure that your mould/aid is correctly inserted.

2 Check that your mould is undamaged.

3 Check whether the tube is blocked by wax or moisture.

4 Consider whether a visit to the audiologist is required to check the function of the aid and/or take an impression for a new mould.

Distortion of sound

Sounds may appear to be distorted when you first use your aid. This can be due simply to unfamiliarity, or perhaps you have the volume too high in an effort to hear more, or it could be that the aid is inappropriately adjusted. Unfortunately an element of distortion is common in particular types of hearing loss such as that associated with Meniere's disease and some sensorineural losses, in which case it can be difficult to resolve because it is a feature of the loss, not the result of a malfunctioning aid. If the fault is with the aid, however, try the following solutions:

1 Paradoxically turning your aid down slightly can reduce distortion and improve the quality of the sound you hear.

2 If you are a new hearing aid user and the problem persists after a four-week trial period or is sufficiently bad to prevent you using your aid, a visit to the audiologist is required.

3 A visit to the audiologist may also be needed if the distortion arises suddenly. In such a case your aid may well be faulty.

Loud sounds are painful

After even a short period of hearing loss, the world heard through your new aid can seem like a very noisy place. Hence the need for listening practice. Yet it is a feature of some types of hearing loss that sudden loud sounds cause discomfort or distress which is severe enough to limit use of a hearing aid, despite your having tried to get used to amplified sound. If your ears have a reduced ability to deal with loud sounds (sometimes referred to as recruitment), the solutions to this problem are limited:

1 Inform your audiologist. It is possible that adjusting the presets (for example, applying peak clipping) could be the answer.

2 Modifying your mould might also relieve the discomfort, so again visit your audiologist to discuss the problem.

3 You may require a special type of hearing aid to resolve matters. Known as a compression aid, this essentially squashes the sound so that it no longer causes discomfort.

Lack of clarity

Most sounds are loud enough for you to be aware, say, that someone has spoken, but are simply not clear. This may well be due to either an inappropriate or an incorrectly adjusted aid, in which case your audiologist may be able to do something about it. The problem is associated with a sensorineural loss, and a high-frequency loss in particular: your ear has lost the ability not only to hear but also to process high-pitched sounds, resulting in what is known as reduced speech discrimination. But even though it is a problem that can rarely be resolved completely by adjusting or changing your aid, it is possible to improve matters:

1 See your audiologist for a hearing aid check. Modern technology such as the REMS machine, if available, will enable him or her to decide if your aid is giving you the full range of sounds necessary to hear speech clearly.

2 Speechreading (lipreading) – that is, learning to use the visual aspects of speech to supplement the sounds you hear – will help.

3 Developing tactics such as making sure that your attention has been drawn to the speaker before he or she begins to speak will help enormously.

Poor sound quality

It is not unusual to feel that sounds through your aid are tinny or too sharp at first. If you have not been hearing the higher-pitched sounds of speech ('sh', 't' and so on) for some time, you are really going to notice them when wearing your aid. These sounds are very important to your understanding of speech, so while they may be rather irritating initially it is important that you try to get used to them again – which you will. But if the problem persists or is preventing you from using your aid, you must seek the help of your audiologist. Solutions include the following:

1 Adjusting the tone controls of an aid can alter how it responds to sound and possibly reduce tinniness.

2 Use of filters is sometimes an option.

Background noise

Perhaps your aid is wonderful one to one, but as soon as there is any background noise you are struggling. It is probably safe to say that this is the most common complaint made by wearers of hearing aids, yet unfortunately it is also the most difficult to rectify. The reasons for this are complex but basically boil down to the nature of sound and the limitations of current technology. Background noise can be a problem for the normally hearing person as well, but is particularly annoying for you because your aid is only an amplifier of sound and it amplifies everything – your companion's speech as well as the hubbub of others in conversation and the almost ever-present music.

So why can't your aid simply amplify the speech and not the background noise? The reason is that they are one and the same: that is, complex sounds made up of lots of different puretones or frequencies. When you reduce the amount of low-frequency sound your hearing aid produces in an effort to get rid of the background noise, this also affects the amount of low-frequency speech sounds you can hear. And as the world we live in is a very noisy place, completely eliminating background noise from every part of your life would be impossible. Coping with background noise will involve compromises with advantages in some situations balanced by disadvantages in others. Here are some solutions you can try:

1 It is possible that altering the aid's frequency response using tone controls may improve matters. You and your audiologist will therefore need to experiment to find the best settings for your lifestyle.

2 Reducing background noise – for example, turning the television off or down – can make an enormous difference to how much you will

Practical advice on coping with a hearing loss

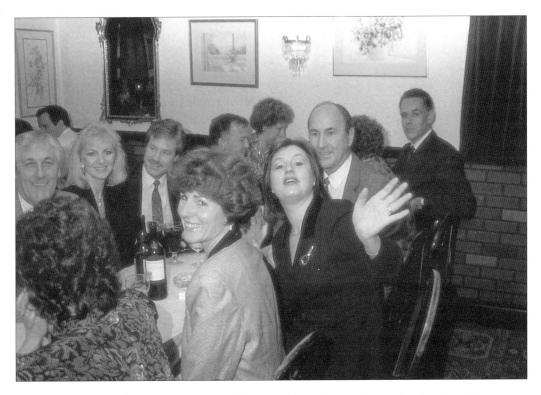

Background noise is the most common problem experienced by people wearing hearing aids.

hear of, say, a mealtime conversation. Dealing with this problem is covered in more detail under 'Communication tactics' (page 45).
3 Improving your ability to use the visual aspects of speech will help in those situations where noise is inevitable.
4 Altering the ear mould may help, although this is not feasible for severe hearing loss.

Discomfort and irritation

There is no doubt that wearing an aid for the first time can feel odd, but it should not be at all uncomfortable. Give yourself time to learn how to put it in properly and to get used to having it there. This can take a few weeks, but if discomfort still persists or is sufficient to stop you from using your aid, see your audiologist straight away, because wearing an aid need not be an uncomfortable experience. Physical discomfort is usually due to a badly fitting mould or casing and can be improved very easily by either filing the mould to fit better or making a new one.

Wearing your aid may cause your ear to feel warm and slightly itchy at first, but your skin will become accustomed to being in close contact with the mould. If, however, this continues and worsens or is accompanied by irritation such as reddening, flaking of the skin in your ear or production of moisture, you should discontinue use of the aid and seek your doctor's opinion: you may have either an allergy to the mould material or an infection which requires treatment. Ear moulds can be made of different materials including hypoallergenic kinds with or without colouring, so it should be possible to solve an allergy problem.

Courses of action you can take include the following:

1 If you are experiencing severe irritation, visit your doctor to eliminate infection as the possible cause before seeing the audiologist.

2 Have a new mould or casing made.

3 Occasionally a tiny vent through the mould can relieve mild sensations of blockage or prevent the ear from feeling too warm.

4 In extreme cases, such as chronic discharge or unresolved allergy, an alternative form of amplification may have to be considered, such as a bone-conduction aid that does not require a mould to be worn (see page 31).

Communication tactics

You may well be wondering at this point what more you can possibly do to improve matters. After all you now wear your aid regularly and have an amplified telephone, a flashing alarm clock and a loop for your television. However, despite all your best efforts, coping with your loss and its effects on your daily life is still a bit of a battle, leading you to opt out more often than you would truly like to. Refusing, say, an invitation to try a new restaurant is a lot easier than struggling to converse all evening and dealing with the inevitable indigestion afterwards. Yet this really need not be the case, for by using and teaching others in your life a few simple tactics you can improve most communication situations immensely. Let us consider for a moment what can make a meal in a restaurant a miserable experience for you: the hubbub of conversation, background music, waiters clattering to and from the kitchen. You probably think that there is nothing you can do about any of this – not so! Choosing a restaurant that does not have music, sitting at a table away from the kitchen door and seating yourself with your back to a wall or corner facing, as far as possible, all your companions can make all the difference to whether you develop indigestion or not.

In short there are many tactics you can use to ease communication. Some you can adopt yourself; some will necessarily involve others; all will require change of some sort. This is the difficult part, for accepting change is not always easy and old habits certainly do die hard. Because you live with your loss 24 hours a day and understand the limitations of your aid, you are well aware of what you can and cannot hear. So using tactics like ensuring that you are in the same room as another person before you begin a conversation with him or

Practical advice on coping with a hearing loss

her will become second nature very quickly. It will not be as easy for others: if they have normal hearing and can easily hear your 'What did you say?' they will forget that speaking to you through a door is futile. Patience will therefore be needed on both sides and you may have to perfect the art of the gentle but firm reminder! This small scenario illustrates the importance of the fundamental rule for good communication: always face the person you wish to speak to. Besides being the polite thing to do, this small action ensures:

● that you have each other's attention;
● that you can both take full advantage of all the non-verbal clues the human face gives – a smile, a frown, a raised eyebrow;
● that you can utilize all the clues that lip movements provide as words are spoken. Speechreading (lipreading; see page 49) is something most of us do without realizing, particularly those of us with a hearing loss;
● that your words do not drift off into the ether but are directed at the person who needs to hear them to communicate with you.

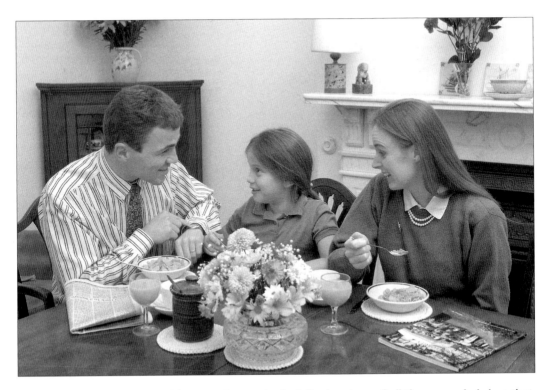

Always face the person you wish to speak to and take full advantage of all the non-verbal clues that face and body can give.

An ideal communication situation would involve two people sitting about 1–2 m/3–6 ft apart in a room with soft furnishings that had virtually no background noise and a good level of lighting, ensuring that they can see each other's face clearly: bliss for anyone wearing a hearing aid and very relaxing for others too, but unfortunately this is not an ideal world. The box below suggests what you can do to help yourself if you have a hearing loss.

What you can do to help yourself communicate more easily

● Wear your spectacles if you need them – an out-of-focus face will be of little or no use to you.

● Remember to switch on your hearing aid. Inform the person to whom you are speaking that you need to see their face.

● Not everyone feels comfortable telling people that they have a hearing loss, so try telling them you wear an aid that helps but that you still need them to speak clearly.

● Try to assess the background noise and reduce it if possible: turning the television off or waiting for the kettle to finish boiling furiously takes time but will make a difference.

● Choose your seat in a group situation so that you can see as many people's faces as possible.

● When joining a group conversation, ask about the topic, if it is not immediately evident. Being aware of the context can make a difference to how quickly you settle into the group.

● Try not to bluff when you have not caught a point or lose the thread as this will only compound your difficulties. Many people with a hearing loss would make excellent poker players because of their highly developed ability to cover up when they have misunderstood! Put the onus back on the speaker by asking for clarification or that they rephrase a sentence. Remember that communication is a two-way process and that you have responsibility for only half of it: the other participant of any exchange can do a lot to help you.

● Allow yourself time out. Give yourself at least half an hour every day when you do not have to use your hearing if you do not want to. Take your aid(s) out and relax, forget about listening to anything, read a book, sit in the garden, have a long hot bath and above all resist the temptation to use your ears. Remember to tell your family beforehand!

Practical advice on coping with a hearing loss

How others can help

We have learnt a great deal about hearing loss in the preceding chapters, but if your hearing is good it is impossible to understand just how frustrating, isolating and depressing not being able to communicate easily can be. A person with a hearing loss can never relax completely because listening is a conscious activity that requires effort. He or she cannot switch off even for a moment during a conversation, since a brief lapse can result in losing the gist completely.

Those who hear well can find it difficult to appreciate that the ability to hear may vary and that some situations are much easier to cope with than others. Therefore it is important to resist the temptation to assume that a person with a hearing loss has some sort of choice in the matter: they do not. Flexibility and an awareness of the needs of people with hearing loss are the keys to maintaining communication.

Considering these facts, it is small wonder that developing a hearing loss can manifest itself with shortness of temper and overwhelming fatigue. However, as a hearing

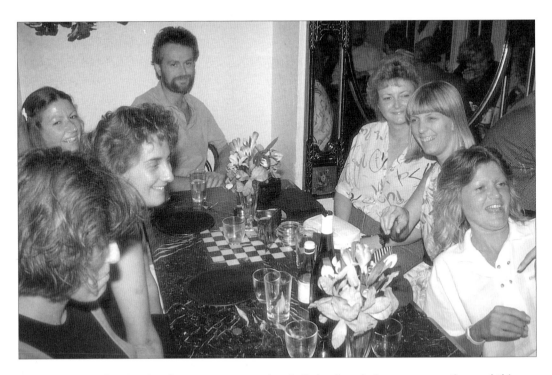

A person with a hearing loss has to concentrate hard all the time during a conversation and this can be very tiring.

person you can do a lot to make communication easier:

● Remember to face the person to whom you are speaking.

● Never shout as this is usually futile – louder is rarely better and it distorts the shape of your mouth.

● Speak clearly at a slightly slower pace but maintaining the natural rhythm of your speech – overmouthing one. . . word. . . every. . . two. . . seconds will not help at all, but it will make you look rather odd while you are doing it!

● Do not chew gum, smoke or cover your mouth with your hands when speaking – obvious, perhaps, but many of us do.

● Rephrase rather than repeat a phrase again and again – sometimes a particular speech sound cannot be heard and no amount of repetition will result in it being heard.

● Remember to stand in the light: your face must not be shadowed, because everything about it adds to communication – your expression, your eyes and, above all, your lips forming the words as you speak.

● Try to be aware of background sounds. Attempting to have a conversation in a noisy street will be a waste of time and energy for all concerned. Reduce background sound if at all possible – choose a quiet venue for an after-work drink; consider whether the television has to be on during the evening meal.

● Try to remember that some rooms make for easier listening than others. Coping with a hearing loss is far easier in a small room with soft furnishings than in a huge bare hall with a high ceiling where sounds simply bounce around.

● Watch the face of the person to whom you are speaking to be as aware of their face as they are of yours. A slightly knotted brow or a quizzical look show clearly that you have failed to communicate something that makes sense. Be sensitive: tutting or saying 'never mind' is probably the worst thing you could do.

Speechreading/lipreading

A few words are necessary on the subject of speechreading, mainly to clear up one of the major misapprehensions about it, namely that it is possible to 'read' every word that can be uttered. This is not the case, if only because a large proportion of English speech sounds are virtually invisible on the lips. Approximately 30 per cent of speech sounds are visible, but unfortunately some of them look exactly the same. P, B and M are an example of this: look at yourself in a mirror and try saying 'pear, bare, mare' without using your voice.

That is not to say that these lipshapes are useless; on the contrary they provide invaluable information to anyone with a hearing loss, which is why it is essential that any conversation is carried out face to face. Learning to speechread is consequently a great deal harder than it first appears because it involves learning to combine knowledge of lipshapes with use of context, and an awareness of body language with an ability to guess and not worry too much about it. This is a skill that comes more easily to certain people, so it is always worth going to a class to develop your abilities – and enjoy the added bonus of meeting others who understand your difficulties.

Chapter five

Coping with tinnitus

The term tinnitus can be traced back to the 17th century, when tinnitus aurium was used to refer to buzzing or tingling in the ears. In fact the condition has existed for at least as long as recorded history, and many famous figures reportedly suffered from it. The painter and sculptor Michaelangelo apparently complained in later life about a racket in his ears and the composer Beethoven is supposed to have commented in his will on the irony of hearing nothing but his tinnitus.

Today the meaning is essentially unchanged – tinnitus simply means noises that are heard in the ears or head for which there is no apparent external source. Tinnitus is commonly called ringing in the ears, but the sound can be anything you care to mention – whistling, hissing, rushing or jangling – provided it does not originate in the environment.

Even if you do not suffer from tinnitus it is very likely that you have had an experience of it along with half the adult population. There are a couple of commonly occurring situations that may well have resulted in your noticing a sound in your ears that did not come from your environment.

For example, can you recall a time when you became aware of a whistling in your ears, perhaps after attending a function with very loud music? This is a very common experience – you probably found that your tinnitus was transitory, disappearing after a period of time lasting anything from minutes to days. Exposure to excessive noise can undoubtedly cause hearing loss and tinnitus in some people, and as it is impossible to predict who will be affected either temporarily or permanently, it is sensible to protect your ears against it. For more information on this topic see 'Protecting your hearing' on page 58.

Have you ever entered a soundproof room or an artificially quiet environment and become aware of hearing something in the silence? If this has happened to you, it was a form of tinnitus that is perfectly normal: the human body is not silent; many of the organs, as they function naturally, produce 'physiological noise' and your ears are no exception. Under normal circumstances you are unaware of intrinsic noises because everyday sounds mask them, preventing you from hearing them.

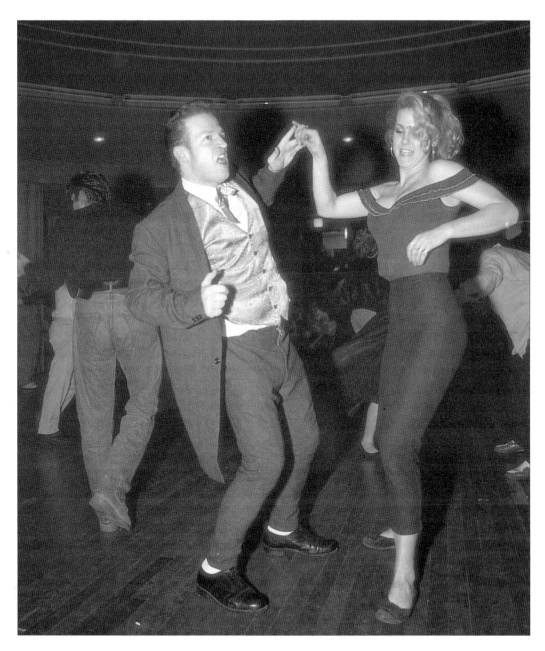

It is not unusual to experience temporary tinnitus after hearing very loud music.

Coping with tinnitus

Facts about tinnitus

- It is a symptom that can have many causes, 99 per cent of which are not sinister, so developing tinnitus does not herald a serious or life-threatening illness.
- It is often associated with hearing loss. However, it is possible to suffer tinnitus without a loss, and developing tinnitus does not necessarily lead to hearing loss.
- It is extremely common. As many as one in four or five adults will experience tinnitus of some sort at some point in their lives.
- More than 85 per cent of people with tinnitus are not bothered by it – it is thought that this is because a natural process called habituation occurs which means they do not pay attention to their noise. This enables them to live with it and prevents it from becoming annoying.
- One in 200 people with tinnitus are significantly troubled by the condition and report that it has a detrimental impact on their daily life. This may manifest itself in a variety of ways such as difficulty in hearing, sleep disturbance, increased irritability, increased sensitivity to everyday sounds, difficulty in concentrating or reduced ability to cope with daily life in general. It is possible with help and support to learn to cope with tinnitus rather than suffer from it and to overcome many of the difficulties mentioned.
- It is more prevalent in the over-45s, so is regarded by some as a natural consequence of the passage of time and the general wear and tear that this imposes on the whole auditory system.
- It can rarely be cured and as yet there is no safe and effective drug treatment available, but as a general rule tinnitus is far more likely to become less noticeable with time than to grow worse. It is possible to learn to live with the condition because it is natural for a process of habituation to occur, although this can take time.

In the light of the facts about tinnitus and the possibility that your reason for reading this chapter is not simply curiosity but because you are possibly struggling to cope with the condition yourself and with the effect it is having on your life, the aims of this chapter are threefold. It aims to achieve the following:

- to answer some of the questions you may have about tinnitus by describing what can cause it and what habituation is;
- to describe some of the methods used to manage tinnitus and the treatment options available;
- to suggest ways you can improve your capacity to cope with tinnitus in your day-to-day life.

The nature of tinnitus

The physiological process that actually produces tinnitus has yet to be fully elucidated and many theories abound, but it is clear that a malfunctioning cochlea plays a part in its development. As already explained, the cochlea is responsible for producing sensory signals which are relayed to the brain via the auditory pathway to be interpreted as sound. If the function of the cochlea is disrupted, this can result in the generation of a stream of irregular or abnormal signals that the brain interprets as sound, which, in the absence of an external source of input, is tinnitus.

What can cause tinnitus?

As in the case of hearing loss, many things can cause tinnitus, some of which are more common than others. Again, as with hearing loss, it is sometimes possible to pinpoint the cause: for example, perhaps you had a bout of flu at the time of the onset. Often, however, the cause cannot be identified and this can be both disappointing and frustrating, particularly if you sought the help of your family doctor, anticipating a diagnosis followed by treatment. It is likely that even if you know the cause of your tinnitus, a cure is remote, but you do not have to live with the way it is making you feel at the time when you consult your doctor, which may well be in some distress. Help is available and your family doctor should at the very least be able to offer reassurance that:
- tinnitus rarely gets worse;
- develop the ability to ignore it;
- he or she can arrange a referral to an

appropriate specialist.

It is not unusual to be worried that tinnitus is a harbinger of something serious, so a referral to an otolaryngologist should allay any fears. Increasingly otolaryngologists with an interest in tinnitus are setting up special clinics that offer the services of a multidisciplinary team of professionals. The team may include hearing therapists, audiologists and psychologists offering a variety of treatment options such as counselling, cognitive therapy, the provision of maskers or white noise generators and relaxation training to tinnitus sufferers seeking help (see pages 55–7).

The following is a list of some of the possible causes of tinnitus:
- Exposure to loud noise (by far the commonest).
- Ageing of the auditory system.
- Trauma to the ear or head.
- Viral infections (it is common to be able to relate onset to a bout of flu).
- Certain drugs. If you have any concerns about medication you are taking, always consult your family doctor.
- Wax in the outer ear or a middle ear infection, both of which can be dealt with and treated respectively.
- Certain conditions such as Menière's disease (a condition of the inner ear associated with recurrent bouts of dizziness, tinnitus and fluctuating hearing loss) or otosclerosis (a disease which affects the bones of the middle ear, causing a conductive hearing loss; this may be treated surgically).

Coping with tinnitus

What is habituation?

You have five senses, hearing, sight, smell, touch and taste, that provide you with a constant stream of information about your body and your immediate environment. All the information you receive is being processed, but it is literally impossible for you to pay attention to everything that you are feeling, seeing and hearing at any one moment in time. So it is completely normal to cease to pay attention or habituate to information which is constant, such as the sensation of pressure from the chair on which you are sitting or repetitive sounds like the ticking of a clock. While it is possible to perform more than one action simultaneously – driving your car while engaged in conversation, for example – you normally pay attention to just one thing at a time. That can be whatever you are concentrating on: the conversation or information that captures your attention because it is either surprising or important, such as a dog darting into the road in front of you!

Why describe this process in a chapter on tinnitus? Because it goes some way towards explaining why the vast majority of people with tinnitus learn to live quite happily with the condition. They no longer attend to it because they have gone through the process of deciding that it is a sound in their ear or head that has no significance and consequently is to be ignored. It is a natural process, but can take time and this will obviusly vary from person to person – anything from three to possibly 18 months, even if nothing interferes. A number of factors can interfere with the habituation process: for example, you may have a type of tinnitus which is unpredictable, or suffer a high level of anxiety or have other negative feelings about it. The next section suggests ways to obtain help if you are having difficulty dealing with your tinnitus. You will learn that a variety of methods can be used to facilitate the process of habituation and ease the burden of living with what can, for some people, be a distressing condition.

Finding help

Developing tinnitus can be a worrying experience, one that may already have led you to seek a medical opinion either from your family doctor or from a specialist. It is to be hoped that this resulted in any fears you may have had about the cause being allayed by a combination of medical examination and tests. But the nature of tinnitus is such that your doctor may not have been able to offer very much in the way of active medical treatment other than:

- reassurance that you do not have a serious illness or have been imagining your noise;
- information about your tinnitus;
- advice on coping with it;
- referral to an appropriate professional for further help with any distress you may be experiencing as a result of the tinnitus;
- suggesting the trial of a hearing aid if tests reveal a hearing loss;

● arranging for the provision and trial of a tinnitus masker or white noise generator;
● providing information on associations and self-help groups.

Hearing aids and maskers

Hearing aids If the tests performed by your doctor revealed a hearing loss, you might be advised to try a hearing aid. This is because the less you hear of external sounds, the more you are likely to be aware of your tinnitus. A hearing aid should always be fitted by an audiologist or qualified dispenser.

Maskers or white noise generators If you are having difficulty coping with tinnitus, your reaction to the suggestion that you try a device which produces a sound all of its own might strike you as somewhat odd – until the basic rationale has been explained to you. We are all aware that some sounds mask others: for instance, the noise of traffic in a busy street can easily drown out a voice. Similarly you have probably noticed that you are less aware of your tinnitus when you are in an environment with background noise.

A tinnitus masker provides a portable source of sound that usually takes the form of wide-band noise, often described as 'shushing', which can be controlled. It is possible to use a masker in a number of ways:
● as a masker, with the volume of the sound set at or slightly above the level of the tinnitus;
● as a partial masker, with the volume set at a level below the level of your tinnitus so that you listen for the masking sound rather than the tinnitus;
● as a white noise generator worn for six to 16

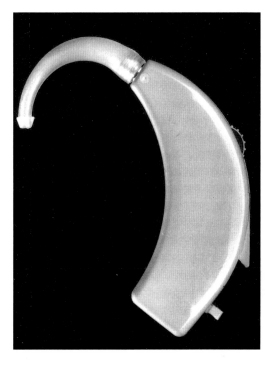

A behind-the-ear tinnitus masker.

hours a day following a programme which can result in reduced awareness of your tinnitus.

A tinnitus masker should always be fitted by an audiologist, therapist or dispenser with appropriate training and experience, preferably in conjunction with supportive counselling as this is crucial to gaining maximum benefit from its use.

The psychological approach

Tinnitus is a physical condition that can cause psychological distress if the natural process of habituation is inhibited in any way. A number of factors can slow down the process: for example, a high level of anxiety or tension

Coping with tinnitus

which may be due to the tinnitus itself or to other stresses. It is not uncommon for tinnitus to be first noticed or developed at a time of great stress such as a bereavement. How you feel about your tinnitus can also affect your ability to cope with it. If you are angry that you developed it after a procedure such as ear syringing, it is likely that you will continue to pay attention to it until your anger recedes. The psychological treatment of tinnitus often hinges on reducing your level of tension and this can be achieved in a number of ways, including relaxation training, cognitive therapy and counselling.

Relaxation training
Learning a method of relaxation can break the cycle of increased tension/awareness of tinnitus/increased tension, because in theory it is not possible to be stressed out and relaxed at the same time.

Cognitive therapy
Cognitive therapy is a widely practised form of psychotherapy that aims to change the way you feel about your tinnitus by changing the way you think about it. Discussions can help put the tinnitus in perspective, enable you to think more positively and learn not to respond

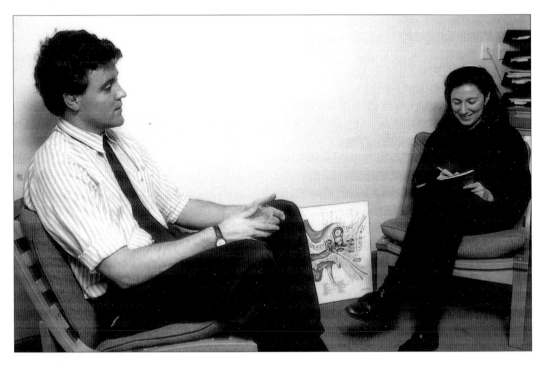

A counselling session with a clinical pshychologist.

to your noises. It can be challenging and hard work, but can result in your coping more easily with your tinnitus. Your specialist may be able to refer you to a psychologist for treatment.

Counselling

Counselling is a less formal treatment than cognitive therapy and may be more readily available. Most people, whatever their problem, benefit from talking to someone about it. However, it is important that the counsellor has an appropriate professional background and some understanding of tinnitus and hearing loss. If you are able to obtain a referral to a specialist tinnitus clinic, it is likely that a number of different professionals will be able to provide counselling – the doctor, the audiologist or a hearing therapist.

Associations and self-help groups

Where can you go for further information? National tinnitus associations exist in most countries and a number are listed at the end of this book on pages 78–9. The services these organizations provide can vary, but most have an information service that collates and disseminates details of local groups as well as keeping abreast with and sometimes funding research and much much more.

Self-help groups are an option and although they do not appeal to everyone they do have a place, because many people value being in contact with others who know what it is like to have a particular condition such as tinnitus. Details of local groups are sometimes advertised in the local press and lists are often available from the national associations.

Developing your strategies

It is hoped that the strategies and ideas outlined below will enable you to cope more easily with your tinnitus.

Solving a sleep problem

Tinnitus at night presents a particular problem or set of problems, because it can be difficult at this time to use distraction and/or masking techniques to full effect. Invariably the level of environmental masking noise is reduced and it is not always appropriate or desirable to replace it with, say, a radio on low volume, although this is an option. You can, however, try the following strategies to help yourself:

● Do not go to bed until you are tired.

● Buy a relaxation tape or learn a relaxation technique and establish a relaxing pre-bed routine such as taking a warm bath or having a hot drink or a nightcap.

● Try not to think about going to sleep or the day's activities but imagine a pleasant and positive image.

● Purchase a pillow speaker and a tape player so that you can listen to your chosen masking sound without disturbing others.

● Try a blocking technique: repeat a word or sound by saying it without sound rather than just thinking it.

● Discuss your sleep problem with your family doctor if you feel you need further help.

Coping with tinnitus

Making the most of masking

Masking works for a number of reasons. It has an external source; it can be modified, controlled and turned off at will; and it can be tailored to a certain extent to be a pleasing sound if required. When and how you use masking will depend largely on whether it is a strategy that works for you and at what times your tinnitus is troublesome. Perhaps it bothers you only when you are trying to read, so you have not considered using masking but have given up reading instead. Using low-level masking may well allow you to enjoy reading again. Remember that masking means using an external sound to cover up your tinnitus, so it can be any sort of sound. If your tinnitus is a problem when, say, you are trying to relax at work during your lunch break because the office is quiet, go for a stroll and listen for environmental sounds to mask your tinnitus.

Distraction

Activities that absorb your attention will prevent you dwelling on or listening to your tinnitus. Take up a hobby, go to that evening class that you have been thinking about for months. As with masking, distraction is a strategy that is useful in itself and when used in conjunction with others.

Engaging the support of family and friends

This is a strategy that can make living with tinnitus much easier. Others may not be aware that your increased irritability in the evenings is due to the fact that you find your tinnitus harder to cope with when you are tired and stressed after work. Try 15 minutes of relaxation time listening to a favourite piece of music before joining the family for the evening meal.

Protecting your hearing

During the course of this book we have learnt that exposure to excessive noise can result not only in the development of tinnitus but also in a hearing loss – intense sound can damage the sensitive structure of the cochlea. A noise-induced hearing loss tends to manifest itself as a drop in the ability to hear the high frequencies (around 4–8kHz), but it will spread to other frequencies if exposure continues.

What constitutes excessive noise?

It is difficult to define excessive noise because the amount of sound an individual can take

before he or she develops a noise-induced loss or tinnitus depends upon a number of factors such as age, susceptibility and previous exposure. Any sound that causes a temporary drop in hearing or a bout of tinnitus is too loud. If, for instance, you have ever left a concert feeling that your hearing was muffled, it was too loud for you. Similarly if using a drill to put up a shelf made your ears ring, it was too loud for you. The only way to cure tinnitus or hearing loss caused by noise is to prevent it in the first place, so it is sensible to take precautions.

Taking precautions

Most developed countries have introduced regulations that require employers to take action if noise exceeds certain levels. This normally involves either limiting exposure time or reducing the level of the sound. So if you are exposed to noise in the workplace, at the very least you should be given the opportunity to wear ear plugs and ear defenders to reduce the level of sound.

This is a sensible policy to adopt as a general principle, without going to the extreme of avoiding loud sounds altogether. If you play in a band, wear musician's ear plugs. Buy a pair of ear defenders to use with noisy household DIY equipment. Avoid sitting directly in front of music speakers at social occasions where the level of sound means you have to raise your voice to be heard.

In the USA the National Institute on Deafness and other Communication Disorders (NIDCD) of the National Institutes of Health has recently instigated a campaign which focuses on educating children at an early age about the potential risks of loud noise. It takes the form of a teacher's guide and a videotape called 'I Love What I Hear' that will be distributed to elementary and middle schools throughout the USA. The purpose of the video is to teach children aged eight to 11 years to conserve their hearing by encouraging them to protect themselves from a variety of potentially harmful environmental sounds such as gunfire, power tools, loud music and engine noise. It is a campaign that the NIDCD hopes will be adopted by other countries.

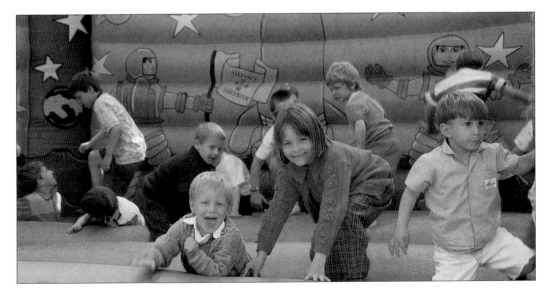

It is important to make children aware at an early age of the dangers of exposure to excessive noise.

Chapter six
Children with hearing loss and deafness

The topic of hearing loss and deafness in children is so expansive that it is not possible to do more than scratch the surface in this chapter. However, it does include a brief look at the causes of hearing loss and deafness in children as these vary a little from the causes of loss in adults. A consideration of some of the signs that can indicate a hearing problem follows, and a natural adjunct to this is recognizing that management of a conductive hearing loss, very common in childhood, may require particular strategies.

Hearing loss acquired in adulthood can undoubtedly have an impact on communication because it interferes with ability to hear spoken language, our main means of communicating. A loss developed very early in life can affect the acquisition of language which is essential for effective communication, so early recognition of the existence of a loss is essential. Some of the methods used to determine whether a child has normal hearing or not are detailed on page 66.

Of course, language need not necessarily be spoken. Deaf people and their communities using sign language are testament to this fact.

Terminology

For the purpose of this chapter the words deaf and deafness will be used to refer to children with a profound or total loss of hearing (that is, no recordable response to a puretone at 96dBHL). It is possible to use a variety of terms to describe a person with a hearing loss which is less than total, for instance:
- partially hearing;
- partially deaf;
- hearing impaired;
- hard of hearing.

However, the wisest course is always to be guided by the person to whom you are speaking – it is a matter of personal choice how someone with a hearing loss wants to refer to themselves or their loss.

With the proper support, encouragement and education it is possible for profoundly deaf children who are unable to utilize amplification to learn a language that permits effective

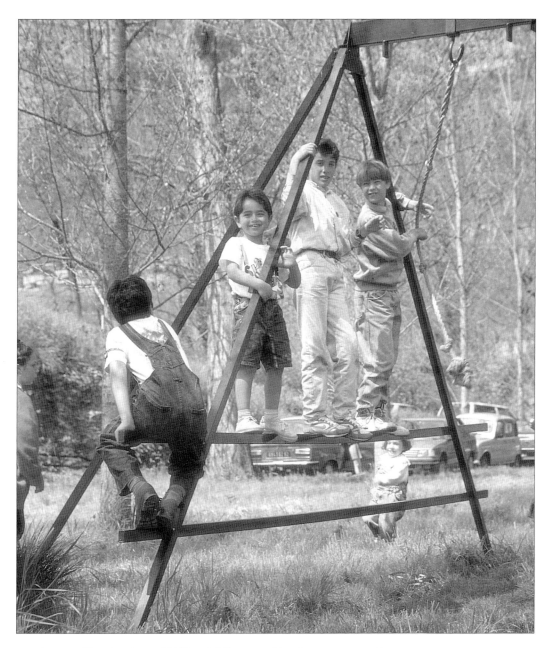

No degree of hearing loss will kill a child's natural instinct to communicate.

Children with hearing loss and deafness

communication and hence allows them to realize their full potential. The issue of language development and what is right for children born with or developing a profound loss before they have acquired language has been the subject of debate for many years.

The urge to communicate is a natural instinct that the existence of a hearing loss of any degree does not quash – a child will always try to communicate. The section entitled 'Communication tactics' suggests ways to facilitate communication at home and at school.

Causes of hearing loss and deafness in children

The causes of hearing loss and deafness in children can be divided into two types: congenital and acquired.

Congenital hearing loss and deafness

Congenital hearing loss and deafness are present at or very shortly after birth. They can be further defined as prelingual because the loss of hearing occurs before language has been developed. It may be the result of:
● an inherited condition (the most common cause);
● German measles (rubella) during pregnancy, now less common in countries with programmes of immunization of schoolchildren;
● prematurity – deprivation of oxygen and neonatal jaundice;
● ototoxic drugs taken during pregnancy;
● cytomegalovirus, for which some countries

have introduced screening programmes;
● rhesus incompatibility.

Acquired hearing loss and deafness

Acquired hearing loss and deafness develop after birth, usually as a result of disease or accident. They can occur before the development of language or after it, in which case they are described as postlingual. Causes include:
● meningitis;
● trauma to the head or ear;
● ototoxic drugs;
● mumps or measles;
● conductive hearing loss as a result of allergy, infection or injury.

However, it is important to bear in mind that it is, as with hearing loss and deafness in adults, more often than not impossible to pinpoint the cause.

Signs and symptoms

An initial piece of advice must be that if you have any concerns at all about your child's

ability to hear, irrespective of his or her age, you should in the first instance consult your

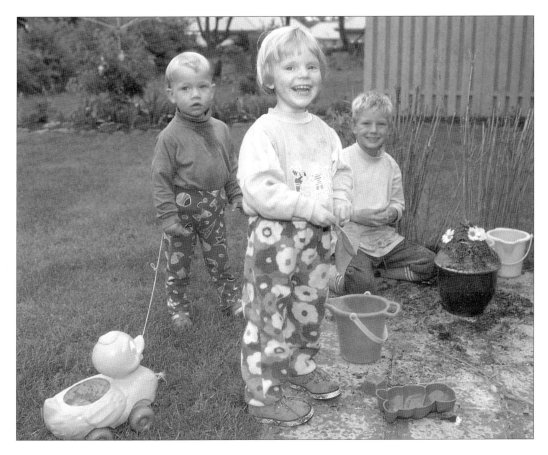

Unfortunately it is often impossible to identify the cause of hearing loss in children.

family doctor. Most countries have instigated screening programmes that aim to detect hearing loss at a very early age, but it is still possible for a child with a hearing loss to fall through the net. However, most professionals working with children recognize that the person caring for the child is the one most likely to be aware of a hearing problem, so do not be afraid to request a referral to a specialist if you are worried in any way. The lists in the boxes on pages 64–5 are not intended to alarm but to provide guidelines that will enable you to decide if you need to seek a further opinion. It is also essential to remember that we are all different, so some children reach milestones faster than others. And older children failing to respond to requests to turn off the television may simply be exhibiting teenage intransigence, not providing evidence of a temporary hearing loss!

Children with hearing loss and deafness

Signs that may indicate the presence of a hearing loss

The under-twos

Birth to six months
- Not responding in any way to a sudden loud sound.
- Failure to imitate sounds.
- No response to noise-making toys.
- Lack of response to your voice.
- Failure to search for a sound with eye or head movements.

Six to ten months
- Does not look for the source of your voice.
- Reduction in production of sounds, no longer babbling.
- No response to a sudden loud sound.

Ten to 15 months
- Showing no response to the sounds of daily life such as the dog barking or the doorbell ringing.
- Loud vocalizations of high-pitched sounds or vowel sounds, 'oohs' and 'aahs'.
- Failure to imitate sounds and lack of attempt to produce words.
- You have to raise your voice to get your child's attention.

The older child

- Inconsistent response to sound.
- Watching a speaker's face very intently.
- Apparent favouring of one ear – tilting head to one side.
- Inability to tell where a sound is coming from.
- Volume of the television higher than is comfortable for others.
- A change in the level of speech – louder or quieter than normal.
- Frequent requests for repetition.
- Inappropriate answers to questions.
- Reports of lack of attention in class.
- Bouts of difficult or unco-operative behaviour.
- Tendency to withdraw or day-dream.
- Tendency to omit certain speech sounds.
- Mispronunciation of words in common usage.

This list is seemingly endless, but a combination of five or six of these signs could very well indicate the existence of a hearing loss, in which case it would be wise to consult your family doctor. Early intervention will prevent later problems.

Symptoms that may be associated with a hearing loss

As with the signs, this list of symptoms is by no means all-inclusive or definitive and should be regarded only as a guide. The presence of one or all of these symptoms does not necessarily confirm the existence of deafness or a hearing loss, but might indicate that you need to consult your doctor if they persist.

- Frequent earache.
- Discharging ears.
- Repeated throat infections.
- Constant copious nasal discharge.
- Itching ears.
- Complaints of noises in the ears.
- Difficulties with balance.

Coping with a conductive hearing loss

In children one part of the human ear in particular is associated with hearing loss: the eustachian tube. This is responsible for maintaining the pressure of the middle ear at a level that permits the efficient transmission of sound to the inner ear. Anything that interferes with the function of the eustachian tube or the middle ear can result in the development of a temporary conductive hearing loss known as glue ear. This is not, of course, the only cause of conductive hearing loss in childhood, but it is extremely common: 20 per cent of all children suffer from it. The reason is that in a child the tube is shorter and wider and points in a more horizontal direction than in an adult, which, in combination with a naturally lower resistance, can allow infection to travel up to the middle ear.

In addition repeated colds, enlarged adenoids or allergies can result in partial or complete obstruction of the tube which is not relieved, as usual, by swallowing. The membrane-lined middle ear produces fluid which is normally liquid and watery that easily drains away down the eustachian tube. If the tube closes, however, the air in the middle ear is gradually absorbed and replaced by the fluid which thickens to form a thin jelly that does not drain easily, resulting in glue ear. The hearing loss may fluctuate and a child with glue ear will not necessarily complain of difficulty hearing, but the loss may manifest itself only as a lack of attention or naughty behaviour. So if your child suffers from repeated colds and bouts of anti-social behaviour, appears not to pay attention on occasion or complains of earache, 'popping', a feeling of fullness or noises in the ear, he or she may be suffering from glue ear.

Children with hearing loss and deafness

Treatments and strategies for managing glue ear

The vast majority of cases of glue ear clear up quite naturally and do not require medical intervention. The ear begins to function normally again of its own accord and the hearing loss is corrected without any further problems. However, some children may require medical treatment if they are particularly prone to bouts of glue ear.

Medical treatment

Medical treatment may involve:
● prescription of antibiotics;
● prescription of nasal decongestants;
● surgical intervention – provision of grommets (a small plastic tube is inserted into each eardrum to allow the 'glue' to drain away, restoring normal function).
● testing for allergies that may be causing the episodes of glue ear.

Strategies for dealing with a fluctuating conductive loss

At school classrooms can be very noisy places and any background noise can make hearing the teacher a problem. Always inform the class teacher that your child has a fluctuating hearing loss and stress the importance of good tactics, such as facing the child when speaking, making sure that he or she is paying attention, that he or she is wearing a hearing aid if one has been provided as a temporary means of dealing with the consequences of glue ear, and that he or she is seated in a position that allows a clear view of the teacher's face.

At home living with a hearing loss can be difficult for the person with the loss and for those in contact with that person. Children with glue ear may exhibit angelic behaviour when they are free of the condition, but suddenly become unmanageable and grossly anti-social when they are unable to hear properly. Tolerance and understanding are all-important if the consequences of this type of hearing loss are not to be permanent.

If your child has to have grommets inserted, your specialist will explain the procedure in detail and discuss any queries you have.

Methods of diagnosis in children

It is possible to determine whether a child has a hearing loss solely from behavioural observation, but this takes time and relies totally on the expertise of the observing professional. Other methods are now available, for example:
● **Otoacoustic emissions (OAEs)** See the glossary (page 77) for an explanation of the theory behind this test. It is non-invasive and can easily be utilized as a means of screening newborn babies with a family history of hearing loss or those exposed to factors that may predispose them to hearing loss or deafness.
● **Brain stem evoked response (BSER)** This test, also described in the glossary, is used to diagnose the presence of a deficit in hearing in babies and small children as well as in adults. It is an objective test that does not require active participation on the part of the person being tested, but provides only limited information about the type of hearing loss.
● **Distraction test** When a baby is physically

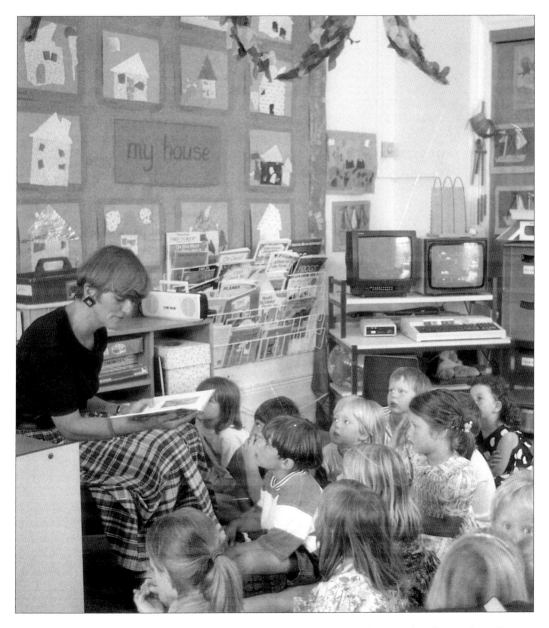

It is very helpful if the class teacher can ensure that the child with a hearing loss has a clear view of his or her face.

Children with hearing loss and deafness

able to move its head in response to a stimulus such as a sound, it is possible to use distraction testing to determine whether it has a hearing loss. This method depends upon the natural response of a child to hearing a sound which is to turn towards it. It is also a method of testing that relies heavily on the expertise of the professionals performing the procedure and the calibraton of the equipment used. But it can result in the early diagnosis of the presence of a hearing loss or deafness.

● **Play audiometry** As the name implies, this type of hearing test depends upon the urge of children to play and to some extent on how readily they respond to being conditioned to react to a sound. It is a subjective test that relies totally on the co-operation of the small person involved. Your child will be encouraged to place a block or toy in a container in response to a sound, effectively establishing the basis for puretone audiometry if required later in life.

● **Tympanometry** This test involves automatic examination of the middle ear using a probe which painlessly applies differing air pressure to the eardrum. The results can indicate the presence of a conductive hearing loss.

Ultimately it may be necessary to use a combination of tests over a period of time to substantiate the existence of a hearing loss and establish the level of it. This type of loss may be amenable to treatment.

Communication tactics

Effective communication strategies are those that suit the needs of the person who is deaf or has a hearing loss; in other words, they should be tailored to the individual. What suits one person will not suit another – it has to be a matter of choice, but there are a number of general strategies that can be employed in the classroom and at home to ease some of the common difficulties children experience as a result of their hearing loss or deafness. Limitation of space prevents participation here in the ongoing debate on oralism *versus* manualism *versus* total communication, but it is possible to offer suggestions of tactics that can be employed to promote good communication at school, if your child is not attending a school for deaf children and at home, although much of this has been covered in Chapter four.

At school

Does your child's school realize that:
● A hearing loss can cause your child to miss important instructions?
● Following group discussions is bound to be difficult for your child, even if he or she uses a hearing aid?
● Wearing a hearing aid in background noise can be difficult, so minimizing this noise is desirable if at all possible: for example, carpeting can help?
● Living with a hearing loss can be tiring, so coping with difficult subjects late in the school day may mean that full potential is not met?

● Your child may feel isolated by his or her hearing loss or by having to wear hearing aids, so it is important not to draw attention to either?

● The hearing loss may require that your child be given preferential treatment in terms of seating so that he or she is able to see the teacher at all times?

● It may be necessary for the level of hearing loss to be taken into consideration during an oral examination?

At home

For the most part the strategies that should be employed in the home to facilitate communication are dealt with in Chapter four, but a few points can be reiterated here:

● Living with a hearing loss or deafness can be hard – communication is a two-way street and both parties must make an effort. This might mean learning another means of communication such as sign language or maximizing communication tactics such as speaking clearly or rephrasing: be prepared to try these.

● It may be necessary to devise different ways of dealing with every-day communication situations – assistive devices such as a Minicom (see page 36) might be needed.

● Adjusting to and accepting a hearing loss or deafness can take time and you may need help with the process. Help is available from various sources, so consult your family doctor and insist on a referral to a paediatrician with an interest in deafness or a specialist with a multidisciplinary team of professionals such as speech and language therapists and teachers of the deaf.

Chapter seven
New developments

We live in an age when advances in technology often seem to outstrip our ability to assimilate them. Let's be honest: do you really know the function of every key on your video control? In the light of the enormous leaps being made it is not unreasonable to expect that someone somewhere has invented the perfect hearing aid, the aid that cuts out all background noise and amplifies only the sounds you want to hear at the best possible quality. Unfortunately this is not yet the case, but scientists and manufacturers of hearing aids are working towards that goal.

This chapter describes some of the recent developments that are currently available in some countries such as cochlear and bone-conduction implants and looks at some of the more unusual aids such CROS and BICROS systems, deep canal aids and vibrotactile devices.

Cochlear implants

We have learnt during the course of this book that hearing aids can only aid the hearing you have left – so is there a device or aid that can help if you lose all your hearing? Indeed until the late 1970s early 1980s there was little on offer apart from possibly vibrotactile devices (see page 74 for more information) combined with improving speechreading skills. This period heralded the development of the cochlear implant, a device which produces sensations of sound by electrical stimulation of the auditory nerve. This important advance offers hope to some of those people who are unable to benefit from any form of conventional amplification because they have acquired a complete sensorineural hearing loss.

In a normal ear sound waves are converted into a sensory signal that is relayed by the auditory nerve to the brain to be interpreted as sound. A cochlear implant bypasses the part of the ear that no longer functions by directly stimulating the auditory nerve to produce signals which are also relayed to the brain. It would be a mistake to assume that the implant can produce a sensation of sound that is identical to normal hearing – as yet that is not possible. But a person using an implant can, with training, use the sounds provided by the device in three main ways:

● to supplement their speechreading skills;

● to monitor the volume and quality of their voice production;

● to develop increased awareness of environmental sounds.

Many types of cochlear implant are available throughout the world, but at a basic level they all consist of a receiver (microphone) to pick up sounds that are sent to a speech processor, then on to a transmitter which passes the signal to another receiver (usually under the skin behind the ear) to be converted into an electrical signal for transmission to the implanted electrode. The electrode, which may be intracochlea (inserted in the cochlear as shown in the diagram below) or extracochlear (resting on or just inside the oval window), stimulates the auditory nerve which sends signals to the brain to be interpreted as sound. The complexity of the signals sent to the brain depends upon another feature of the electrode: that is whether it is a single-channel or multi-channel device.

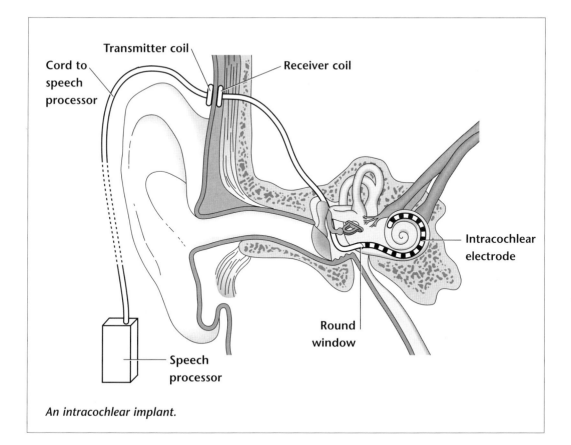

An intracochlear implant.

New developments

Not everyone with a complete hearing loss is a suitable candidate for an implant and indeed not everyone would want one. A number of criteria must be satisfied before anyone can be considered for an implant and these vary from implant programme to programme and from country to country. Initially implants were available only to adults, but since the late 1980s an increasing number of children have been implanted and this has inevitably led to a revision of the basic criteria. One of the main criteria has been that the loss had to have been acquired after the development of speech. The current philosophy regarding the implantation of children is that as early as possible produces the best results. The criteria listed below are therefore only a representation of the original set which had to be satisfied before an adult would be considered for a cochlear implant:

● Profound deafness in both ears.
● Minimal or no benefit from powerful hearing aids.
● Hearing loss acquired after the development of speech.
● Healthy middle ear; no active infection of any kind.
● Good physical fitness; ability to tolerate a general anaesthetic.
● Psychological stability.

Implantation requires surgery to place the electrode and the receiver in the correct position. This can take between two to five hours, with recovery from the surgery in approximately a week.

It must be pointed out here that cochlear implants are not the panacea for everyone with a complete hearing loss/deafness. Many deaf people involved in the established and thriving deaf communities that exist in most countries do not recognize deafness as a disability. This is because they have a rich language and culture, and often the only difficulties they face are the result of ignorance and lack of awareness on the part of hearing people. Moreover there is an element within the deaf community that is opposed to the principle of implantation, and in particular the implantation of children born with a severe to profound hearing loss, partly because of the belief that it denies them the opportunity to become a member of that community. It is virtually impossible even to pretend to address the more controversial aspects of cochlear implants in this book, but it is essential to recognize that controversy does exist.

Bone-anchored hearing aids

It is important to learn a little of the background of these devices because the idea of screwing something into the skull of a person with all its connotations can seem horrifying if not put into context.

When you have a hearing test, the audiologist establishes the level and type of your hearing loss by recording how you respond to puretone sounds first via air conduction using the headphones and second by bone conduction via a small vibrating pad placed on the ridge of bone (mastoid bone) directly behind your ear. A conductive hearing loss is the result of the ear failing to conduct sound to the inner ear. Fortunately a scientist called von Bekesy discovered in 1960 that sounds reaching the inner ear via the bones of the skull were heard in exactly the same way as sounds heard normally. His discovery led to the development of bone-conduction hearing aids, which meant that those people with a conductive loss that could not be helped by surgery or a conventional hearing aid had the chance of hearing well again.

A bone-conduction aid works just like any other hearing aid. Sound received by a microphone is amplified and relayed to the inner ear via the bones of the skull using a small vibrating pad which can be placed on a head band or on the arm of a pair of spectacles and positioned, usually, on the mastoid bone. A disadvantage of this system can be discomfort, because the pad must press quite hard on the bone to transmit the vibration to the inner ear, since the skin covering the bone actually presents quite a barrier to the signal being transmitted effectively. This led to the evolution of the bone-anchored hearing aid which eliminates the problem by having the vibrator screwed directly into the mastoid bone.

Two types of bone-anchored hearing aid are currently in production. Both involve having a minor surgical operation to insert a very small

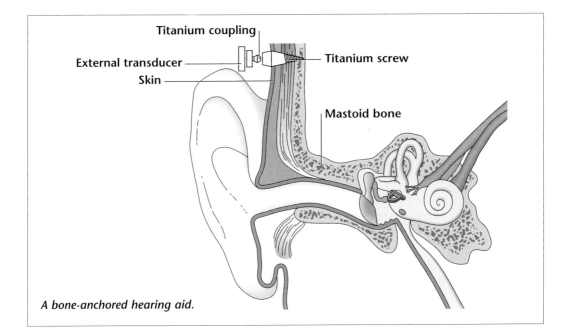

A bone-anchored hearing aid.

New developments

hypoallergenic screw made of titanium into the mastoid bone. Both types also require a small device to be worn externally, but the methods of attachment differ: one uses magnetism; the other plugs directly into the screw. This type of hearing aid is obviously appropriate for only a small number of people for whom

reconstructive surgery is not possible, and for those who cannot use an ear-worn aid. The degree of hearing loss is also a factor which has to be taken into consideration, because the level of amplification these aids provide can help only people with a mild to moderate conductive hearing loss.

Vibrotactile devices

Vibrotactile devices were developed for the benefit of individuals who had lost their hearing completely or were unable to use a conventional aid. Although these devices provide information about sound in the form of vibration, they differ from bone-conduction aids in that they use the sensitivity of the skin rather than the vibration of bone to convey the signal. A number of different types of varying complexity exist, from the single-channel devices, such as the tactile acoustic monitor

(TAM; shown in the photograph below), the Minivib and Minifonator, to the two-channel Tactaid II and the Trill. Sounds are picked up by a microphone which, depending upon the device, is either worn on the lapel or integral to the processor, as in the case of the TAM. The processor then converts the sound into a vibration which is relayed to a small vibrator or tactile stimulator usually worn on the wrist (two in the case of a two-channel device).

It is possible with practice and training to

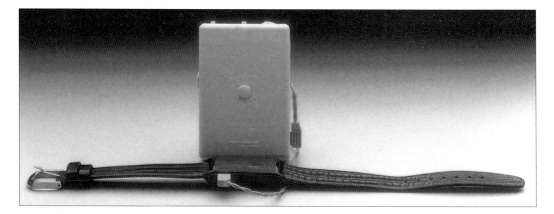

The TAM, a single-channel vibrotactile device. Note the wrist-worn vibrator and the processor.

use a tactile signal to supplement
speechreading skills, although the amount of
information the vibration conveys will depend
upon the way the sound is processed. Some
devices simply convey the rhythm of speech
and some try to produce a vibration that varies
in frequency, enabling the wearer with training
to discriminate between different speech
sounds. Vibrotactile devices also provide an
awareness of environmental sounds and can in
some cases lead to improved speech production
by allowing monitoring of voice level.

CROS and BICROS systems

It is perfectly feasible to cope with most aspects
of daily life with one normally functioning ear
because it is possible to learn to put the
telephone to your good ear and to choose
where you stand or sit in any communication
situation. But because our ears are designed to
work together, a unilateral hearing loss can
sometimes result in difficulties. You rely on
both your ears for your ability to locate a sound
and to tell how far away it is as well as being
able to listen selectively to one sound in the
presence of another. A CROS or BICROS system
could solve the problem of inability to
directionalize and perhaps improve perception
of speech in the presence of another sound.

CROS stands for contralateral routing of
signals. A microphone is worn on the ear that
no longer functions so that sounds are picked
up on that side of the head. The sounds are
then transferred via a wire or radio signal to a
receiver worn on the good ear, and if the
hearing in that ear is normal, the receiver must
be worn with a mould that does not prevent
sounds entering the good ear normally. If the
good ear also has some degree of hearing loss,
it is possible to wear a microphone on each ear
so that amplified sounds from both sides are
fed into the good ear.

As with any form of amplification the
benefits to be gained from a CROS or BICROS
system may not be immediately apparent.
However, with time it is, once again, possible to
pinpoint where a sound is coming from and
manage more easily in a group situation.

Deep canal aids

Hearing aids today are without a doubt a great
deal smaller in general than they were 20 years
ago and the deep canal aid probably represents
the ultimate in discreet devices because it is
virtually invisible. Unlike most in-the-canal
aids it does not protrude from the canal at all,
but is seated deep in the bony part of the ear
canal as shown in the diagram on page 76.

The manufacturers of this type of device
maintain that wax production does not pose a
problem, and the position of the aid in the ear
canal means that sound is heard more

New developments

naturally. The extremely small size of the aid imposes limitations on the components that can be included and consequently this suits only a limited range of hearing losses. The position of the aid in the canal means that the physical shape and condition of the ear canal are very important, so a medical examination is essential before considering acquiring this sort of device. As in the case of any hearing aid an impression of the ear canal has to be taken and with this aid it is necessary for the material to fill the canal completely down to the eardrum. The audiologist performing this procedure must be an expert and extremely careful if no damage is to be done to the eardrum.

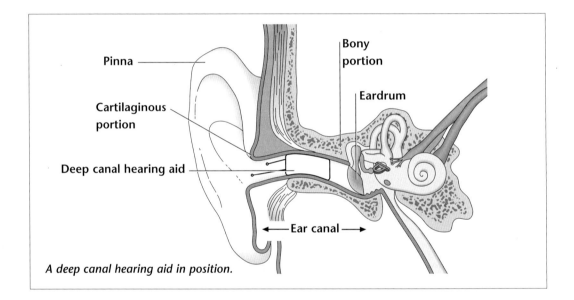

Pinna

Cartilaginous portion

Deep canal hearing aid

Bony portion

Eardrum

Ear canal

A deep canal hearing aid in position.

Research

Research of all sorts into hearing loss is ongoing. In most countries doctors, scientists, audiologists and all the other professionals involved in the field of audiology and the care of people with hearing loss are constantly striving to improve treatments and develop better hearing aids. As well as this they are endeavouring to increase public awareness of the needs of people with hearing loss. Many of the organizations listed on page 78 have information services that enable you to access details of current research and new developments as well as offering all the usual help, so it is always worthwhile making contact.

Glossary

Acoustic neuroma A rare, slow-growing, non-malignant tumour on the eighth nerve (auditory nerve) which may require removal.

Amplitude The physical intensity of a sound equivalent to loudness (the higher the amplitude, the louder the sound).

Bekesy test An automatic hearing test where the threshold of hearing is recorded by an audiometer.

Bilateral Refers to both sides as in, for example, 'a bilateral hearing loss'.

Binaural Refers to both ears as in, for example, 'binaural hearing aids'.

Evoked response audiometry (ERA) Objective tests that are used to assess hearing threshold and establish a diagnosis. For example, electrocochleography (ECochG) and brainstem evoked response (BSER).

Feedback The term used to describe the whistling sound a hearing aid produces if it or the ear mould does not fit properly. A new mould or casing will usually solve the problem.

Frequency Sounds reach the ear as changes of pressure in the air, and this term refers to the rate of these changes and is equivalent to the pitch of a sound.

Hertz (Hz) The international unit of frequency. 200Hz is a low-frequency/low-pitched sound; 6000Hz is a high-frequency/ high-pitched sound.

Hyperacusis An abnormal aversion to or discomfort from sounds that would not normally be regarded as loud.

Otoacoustic emissions (cochlear echo) The sounds a normal cochlea produces in response to receiving an external sound. Their presence is normal and does not contribute to tinnitus; in fact the absence of an echo can indicate a loss of hearing.

Otoscope The instrument the doctor or audiologist uses to examine the ear canal and eardrum.

Presbyacusis This term is often used to refer to a slowly progressing high-frequency hearing loss which is associated with an ageing auditory system.

Real ear measurement system (REMS) Refers to a testing system that enables the audiologist to establish the performance of a hearing aid *in situ* – that is, in the ear.

Recruitment The phenomenon which causes very small increases in sound to be perceived as abnormally loud.

Residual inhibition The reduction in level of tinnitus that can sometimes occur after hearing an external sound that is louder than the tinnitus.

Tinnitus match and mask A test used in some tinnitus clinics to establish the frequency and level of the tinnitus.

'T switch' This feature allows the wearer of a hearing aid to utilize loop systems and inductive couplers.

Useful addresses

British Tinnitus Association (BTA)
Room 6
14/18 West Bar Green
Sheffield S1 2DA
Tel: 01742 796600
Works to combat tinnitus, offers advice and counselling services as well as producing a newsletter that has information on research and tinnitus organizations in other countries.

Royal National Institute for Deaf People (RNID)
105 Gower Street
London WC1E 6AH
Tel: 0171 387 8033
Fax: 0171 388 2346
Minicom: 0171 383 3154
Represents the needs of deaf, deafened, hard-of-hearing and deafblind people and provides a range of services including communication support, training, information and specialist telephone services.

Hearing Concern (formerly the British Association of the Hard of Hearing: BAHOH)
7/11 Armstrong Road
London W3 7JL
Tel: 0181 743 1110
Campaigns on behalf of hard-of-hearing people and provides information on hearing loss, speechreading and local groups.

British Deaf Association (BDA)
38 Victoria Place
Carlisle
Cumbria CA1 1HU
Tel: 01228 48844 (voice and Minicom)
Fax: 01228 41420
Aims to advance and protect the interests of the deaf community.

The National Deaf Children's Society (NDCS)
15 Dufferin Street
London EC1Y 8PD
Tel: (Mon–Fri, 1.00–5.00pm)
0800 252380 (Freephone)
Provides information and advice on all aspects of childhood deafness. This includes a pack for families with a child who has been recently diagnosed as deaf.

Hearing Aid Council
Moorgate House
201 Silbury Boulevard
Central Milton Keynes
Bucks MK4 1LZ
Tel: 01908 585442
Holds a register of qualified dispensers of private hearing aids and has disciplinary powers, but does not act on behalf of individuals seeking recompense from a dispenser.

USA

Alexander Graham Bell Association for the Deaf
3417 Volta Place
Washington, DC 20007, USA
Tel: 202 337 5220
Fax: 202 337 8314
Provides information on hearing loss in adults and children as well as collaborating with professionals involved in research and the care of deaf and hard-of-hearing people of all ages.

American Hearing Research Foundation
55 E. Washington Street
Suite 2022
Chicago, IL 60602, USA
Tel: 312 726 9670
Keeps doctors and the public informed of the latest developments in hearing research and education.

American Society for Deaf Children
Suite 307
814 Thayer Avenue
Silver Spring, MD
20910, USA
Tel: 800 942 ASDC
Provides support and information about deafness to families of deaf and hard-of-hearing children.

American Tinnitus Association
PO BOX 5
Portland, OR
97207, USA
Tel: 503 248 9985
Provides information about tinnitus and referrals to local support groups throughout the USA.

Better Hearing Institute
5021-B Backlick Road
Annandale, VA
22003, USA
Tel: 703 642 0580
Fax: 703 750 9302
Offers a wealth of information on hearing loss and has an information line, 800-EAR-WELL.

National Information Centre on Deafness
Gallaudet University
800 Florida Avenue NE
Washington, DC
20002-3695, USA
Tel: 202 651 5051 (voice)
Collects, develops and disseminates information about all aspects of hearing loss and services offered to deaf and hard-of-hearing people.

CANADA

Western Institute for the Deaf
835 Humboldt Street
Room 302
Victoria
British Columbia,
U8V 2Z6
Tel: 416 225 3281

Canadian Coordinating Council on Deafness (CCCD)
294 Albert Street
Suite 201
Ottawa, ONT KIP 6E6
A source of general information and laws re hearing loss.

The Tinnitus Association of Canada
23 Ellis Park Road
Toronto
Ontario, M6S 2VE·
Tel: 416 2253281.

AUSTRALIA

Australian Tinnitus Association Limited
288 Unwins Bridge
Road
Sydenham
New South Wales, 2044
Tel: 0061 23617331

Australian Hearing Services
Head Office
126 Greville Street
Chatswood
New South Wales, 2067
Tel: (02) 412 6800
Fax: (02) 413 1571
TTY: (02) 283 1762
Dedicated to assisting people with a hearing impairment to function effectively and to reduce the incidence of hearing problems in the community.

NEW ZEALAND

New Zealand Tinnitus Association
North Shore Hospital
Milford
Auckland
Tel: 649 486 5359

SOUTH AFRICA

All organizations and associations are required to register with:
The Dept. of Welfare
Private Bag X828
Pretoria, 0001
Tel: 002712 3202130
Fax: 002712 3223702
This is therefore a source of information on all organizations concerned with the deaf, hard of hearing and tinnitus.

South African National Council for the Deaf
Private Bag X4
Westhoven 2142
Tel: 002711 4821610
Fax: 002711 7265873

Index

Praise for *Screen Tests*

"In *Screen Tests*, a voice who both is and is not the author picks up a thread and follows it wherever it leads, leaping from one thread to another without quite letting go, creating a delicate and ephemeral and wonderful portrait of how a particular mind functions. Call them stories (after Lydia Davis), reports (after Gerald Murnane), or screen tests (inventing a new genre altogether like Antoine Volodine). These are marvelously fugitive pieces, carefully composed while giving the impression of being effortless, with a quite lovely Calvino-esque lightness, that are a joy to try to keep up with."

—Brian Evenson

"If Thomas Bernhard's and Fleur Jaeggy's work had a charming, slightly misanthropic baby—with Diane Arbus as nanny—it would be *Screen Tests*. Kate Zambreno turns her precise and meditative pen toward a series of short fictions that are anything but small. The result is a very funny, utterly original look at cultural figures and tropes and what it means to be a human looking at humans."

—Amber Sparks

"Kate Zambreno writes with a winning, gleeful transparency about days and nights spent entranced by literature, film, and her own densely populated imagination. Above all, Zambreno pays attention to her own desire's fluctuations—to attachments, moods, self-constructions, and self-abasements, reconfigured in a series of shadow-box homages to writing as an asymptotic specter. In rhythm-conscious bulletins, streaked with passionate candor, she confirms her vocation as haunter and as haunted."

—Wayne Koestenbaum

"These stories and essays are layered and build as a Goldin-esque slideshow of textual stills that, often through other art and artists' lives, explore the book's central first-person voice as private figure, as public figure, as member of the (abstract) writing 'community,' as mother, as an aging (female) body, as a person who has escaped their idea of nothingness through dedication to and persistence in making work."

—Jen George

"Weird, daring, triumphant."

—Sofia Samatar

SCREEN TESTS

ALSO BY KATE ZAMBRENO

FICTION

O Fallen Angel

Green Girl

NONFICTION

Appendix Project

Book of Mutter

Heroines

SCREEN TESTS

STORIES AND OTHER WRITING

KATE ZAMBRENO

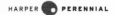
HARPER PERENNIAL

NEW YORK • LONDON • TORONTO • SYDNEY • NEW DELHI • AUCKLAND

HARPER PERENNIAL

HarperCollins books may be purchased for educational, business, or sales promotional use. For information, please email the Special Markets Department at SPsales@harper collins.com.

FIRST EDITION

Designed by Jamie Lynn Kerner

Library of Congress Cataloging-in-Publication Data has been applied for.

ISBN 978-0-06-239204-6

19 20 21 22 23   LSC   10 9 8 7 6 5 4 3 2 1

At the end of my time, when I die, I don't want to leave any leftovers. And I don't want to be a leftover. I was watching TV this week and I saw a lady go into a ray machine and disappear. That was wonderful, because matter is energy and she just dispersed. That could be a really American invention, the best American invention—to be able to disappear.

—ANDY WARHOL

Sometimes I feel I spend my whole life rewriting the same page.

—ANNE CARSON

CONTENTS

ESSAYS
(2012–2014)

SCREEN TESTS

STORIES
(2016–2018)

SUSAN SONTAG

I like to think about what other people do when they're alone. This is what I would really like to know about people, but I never know how to ask. Some people try never to be alone. I once read that about Susan Sontag. That she insisted someone always be with her, when she was eating breakfast, when she was agitating around some idea. I wonder what it would have been like to be Susan Sontag. To exist, in so strong and intense of a mind, the solid outlines of her body. To photograph so definitively, as if there were such a thing as a self. A friend wrote to me recently that she wasn't sure what she thought of Susan Sontag, because if they met, say, at a party, she wasn't sure if she would like Susan Sontag or if Susan Sontag would like her. This was obviously a hypothetical conversation since Susan Sontag has been dead for some time. I liked thinking about that, about how my friend viewed the persona of Susan Sontag, because it was so different from how I thought of Susan Sontag. I don't think of how famous people or people I admire would view me at parties, or if they would recognize something in me if they met me, probably because I do not go to parties, and usually avoid gatherings of more than five people, unless they are book-related gatherings I'm involved in, and then I have no choice. And if I were to think about how I conduct myself at the handful of parties that I have attended in recent years, almost always with fellow writers, I imagine I might not come off too well. I think I might come off as severe, in my dress and in my mannerisms, or if not severe, then formal, or if not formal, then not full of ease, although that's not how I think of myself, or that's only how I think of one version of myself, the writer in public, which might be unconsciously mimicking Susan Sontag. I am actually just pretty awkward because I do not go to many parties, and I'm usually eager to leave. My favorite pastime at a party is studying bookshelves, to see how books are arranged, or not even that, to greet the authors on the shelves as friends. So if Susan Sontag was at a party that I was also at, I would probably be more comfortable going through *Against Interpretation* or *Under the Sign of Saturn* than making small talk with Susan Sontag, for after all, you can tell a lot about a writer by how much Susan Sontag they have on their bookshelf, if they have *Death Kit*, have they read it. Once I think about it, making small talk with Susan

Sontag sounds pretty excruciating. I am pretty sure Susan Sontag would not like me if we met at a party. Perhaps I would be anxious to perform and to say clever things, and I would bring up Michel Leiris and Maurice Blanchot and be unsure as to pronunciation. Maybe Susan Sontag would like me. For me, I don't think it matters. I am sure I would like her, because she is Susan Sontag, and even if she was dismissive or haughty to me, or seemed paranoid and fragile, or brazen and intense, or any of all the adjectives used to describe women like Susan Sontag and even women who are not like Susan Sontag, I think I would appreciate her for it, even love her for it, and know that this was only one version of Susan Sontag, that there were other, private versions of Susan Sontag, Susan Sontag performing to an audience of one, her son or lover or whomever, reading out loud her drafted brilliance, her unbelievable brilliance, and then there is even another Susan Sontag who is completely alone, alone in her thoughts in a comfortable way, or alone in the bathtub, or alone sleeping, or alone in despair, and this, this is another Susan Sontag.

THE FOURTH ANNUAL JEAN SEBERG INTERNATIONAL FILM FESTIVAL

Over a year ago my agent forwarded me an email inviting me to sit on a panel for The Fourth Annual Jean Seberg International Film Festival and to read a new piece of writing on the life and work of Jean Seberg. The press release told me that the festival would take place in late November in Jean Seberg's hometown of Marshalltown, Iowa. I have now found myself on the Wikipedia entry for Marshalltown, Iowa. It seems like a picturesque town with a Main Street. In fact, the first European settler built a log cabin there and called it the "prettiest place in Iowa," much like, I'm imagining, Jean Seberg was also called the prettiest girl in Iowa, or at least in Marshalltown, Iowa. There is a list on the Wikipedia page of Notable People from Marshalltown, Iowa. There are a surprising number of Notable People from Marshalltown, Iowa, in the fields of sports (it's a baseball town), media, civil rights, acting, and politics. I decided to look up my own hometown of Mount Prospect, Illinois, unsure if it has a Wikipedia page. I am somewhat surprised to find that there are several apparently Notable People who were born in the northwest suburb of Chicago where I grew up. A handbag designer I've never heard of who shares my initials and whose bags have been worn by Paris Hilton and Jessica Alba. The television actress Jennifer Morrison. The winner of a season of *American Idol*. Several professional athletes. I spend a moment thinking about the strange category of "success" and its relationship to the other category of "failure," how American these divides are, and how I'm much more compelled lately by the latter, although one cannot be a failure if one does not have at least some image of what success should look like. And that the movement for the Notable People was one of leaving their small towns—they are notable at least in part because they have left Mount Prospect, Illinois, just as Jean Seberg is notable because she left Marshalltown, Iowa. The other day in an existential funk I began to look up online everyone I had gone to high school with whose names I could remember, which was not many people, only to find that most of them have never left; they were all still there, or have moved on to a more upwardly mobile suburb, closer to the Woodfield Mall, like Rolling Meadows, where there's the racetrack and courthouse, or Long Grove, where there's the old-fashioned village of shops. My father, when he speaks of the kids I went to school with, always tells me how many children they have had, and if they're married, because that's his measure of success. Or if they became doctors or lawyers, or perhaps teachers. And yet I must go back to the initial invitation to participate in The Fourth Annual Jean Seberg International Film Festival. I should note that the letter inviting me was specific and knowledgeable about my published work, which has in fact revealed an interest in Jean Seberg, particularly her earlier oeuvre, her work both in *Bonjour Tristesse* and *Breathless*. I realized, reading this invitation, in fact several times, still musing over this invitation now, that I do not know much of what came after these two films for Jean Seberg, and went then as now to her Wikipedia page. There were many points of interest that compelled me—the fact that Jean Seberg was a target of FBI surveillance, much like Marilyn Monroe, and that she was actively involved in the Black Panthers. I was still interested in her early filmography, that she was picked as an unknown to play Joan of Arc by Otto Preminger, and even though the film was a failure, he cast her the next year in *Bonjour Tristesse*. And that even though that film was also a failure, Godard then cast her in *Breathless*, telling her that he wanted her to play the same character as in *Bonjour Tristesse*, that the film could start with the last shot of Preminger's film and then dissolve to a title card that read "Three Years Later." A friend brought up this reference when I was speaking of what I saw as the failure of my last book, which was published several years ago. She said I could just write again some version of the same book, or with the same energy and impulse behind that book. Perhaps all of our books are like that, perhaps we keep on writing toward the same thing, perhaps they could all have a title card that dissolves to read "Three Years Later." When I received the invitation to participate in The Fourth Annual Jean Seberg International Film Festival, I found it enticing, because that is the exact sort of subject matter I like to twist on about—the disappearing acts, the ellipses, the periods of invisibility we cannot know about. Although I should note, the invitation came at a strange time, as I was just, at that moment, having one of those paranoid days spent online, noting that several authors I knew were invited to a literary festival in Australia, including a friend, a more famous novelist. I enjoyed the voluptuousness of it, that I was not ever invited expenses paid to international literary festivals, but I was invited to an international film festival in Marshalltown, Iowa, where I would be given a $150 honorarium, but I would not have my travel and board paid for, as obviously this was a grassroots kind of effort, which I appreciated. I really almost did it. If they had paid a little more, so I didn't have to pay to travel to Iowa, I would have considered it more seriously. Although who am I kidding? I have canceled every event that has involved travel in the past two years, sometimes at the last minute. Was Jean Seberg blackballed by Hollywood for her support of civil rights?

Is it true that the FBI's following of her was responsible for her deteriorating mental health? She is tagged on Wikipedia under "Actresses Who Committed Suicide," "Drug-Related Suicides in France," and "Female Suicides." In the past ten hours an editor at Wikipedia has tried to add her to the more generic and extremely eclectic "List of Suicides," each of which contains a novel someone needs to write (Diane Arbus; Walter Benjamin; John Berryman; Seung-Hui Cho, the Virginia Tech shooter; Gilles Deleuze; Isabella Blow; Yukio Mishima; Alejandra Pizarnik). Seberg's suicide note read, "Forgive me. I can no longer live with my nerves." Her *New York Times* obit headline: "Jean Seberg Found Dead in Paris; Actress Was Missing for 10 Days; A Life of Personal Tragedy." The Wikipedia entry of "Actresses Who Committed Suicide" is extremely long. I feel I've tried to write an essay or poem about half of them at one time or another. Like Peg Entwistle, who leapt from the *H* in the Hollywood sign. Is it worse, I've wondered, the tragedy of the unknown, or the tragedy of the once famous? Edie Sedgwick is not listed, which I find strange. I could spend all day here. When I first received the invitation to The Fourth Annual Jean Seberg International Film Festival, I had been thinking in fact of Edie Sedgwick, of Warhol's Screen Test of her, like a luminous blinking statue staring back at us. It took a while for me to get oriented and realize that I was invited to write about Jean Seberg, not Edie Sedgwick, although for sure, Edie Sedgwick was kind of playing Jean Seberg, she was consciously playing the part, just like Jean Seberg was consciously playing the part from *Bonjour Tristesse* in *Breathless*, or like Candy Darling was consciously playing the part of Kim Novak, or like the cycle of Hollywood actresses on screen self-consciously mimicking the previous history were doubles of the other, like Hedy Lamarr named after Barbara La Marr, or Marilyn Monroe playing a Jean Harlow type, and on and on. I realize now writing this that I never actually replied to my invitation to The Fourth Annual Jean Seberg International Film Festival. Perhaps this will have to suffice. I appreciate the invitation, I do, I would have liked to have taken the time to think more about the life and work of Jean Seberg, I would. I was there in spirit. Yours, et cetera.

BLANCHOT IN A SUPERMARKET
PARKING LOT

There are three elements to the photograph. There is the grocery cart in the background, the white Renault hatchback in the foreground, and then at center there is the reclusive philosopher who explored literature's impossibility. This is one of only three photographs of Blanchot widely known, the other two from when he was much younger. No doubt Foucault was referring to him when saying in an interview that surely there were others like him, who wrote in order to have no face. Amazing to have lived a life and to have authored so many books yet to have avoided being photographed, or having the photographs circulated. Except here, in his fragility, when he probably least expected it. Not even when he resurfaced to support the May 1968 student protests did anyone dare to take his photograph, and now this. The philosopher is nearly eighty years old in this photograph, if it can be called that, as it is more of a paparazzi snapshot, and he is dressed as you might imagine a French intellectual would dress, in a black turtleneck, wool jacket, and thick spectacles. The photograph was published in the June 1985 issue of *Lire*, so he is probably overdressed for the weather. Blanchot most likely didn't have summer clothes. He looks annoyed at this intrusion, and/or annoyed at the indignity of old age and of having trouble getting around. There is something so lonely about the idea of Blanchot going to a supermarket by himself. The monstrosity of the American-style supermarket, all of these options, it can be paralyzing. He will have to carry a brown bag outside himself, or push his cart and load his groceries into his car. What does Blanchot buy at a supermarket? I imagine a list that's ordinary and yet somehow profound, but I struggle to write it. Canned peaches, for some reason, that's what I fixate on. It is impossible to know.

AMAL CLOONEY

Recently, I've noticed that when I google myself, Google states that I am forty-one years old. This bothers me, because even though I am in my forty-first year, I only turned forty-five months ago. Every time I look at this, which is more regularly than I'd like to admit, it bothers me. Why is the Internet aging me so fast? I have been told that this is because my Wikipedia page, which is fairly short and no one has updated in some time, lists the year I was born but not the date. So I'm listed as a "1977 birth." Except I was born on the second-to-last day of the year. I barely count as a "1977 birth," if you really think about it. Since I've turned forty, I've become aware of other women in public who are approximately my age. A friend, a well-known novelist, is almost an entire year older than I am, but we are listed as the same age. She is actually forty-one, however; I am just in my forty-first year. Another famous writer, who dislikes me because of a falling-out a few years ago, is listed as forty because she was born in 1978, but in reality we are less than two weeks apart. I think it's possible I'm this writer's nemesis, although she is not mine. When I first moved to the city and felt alienated by the publishing world, I developed several nemeses, perhaps as a defensive tactic, but since then I have felt too tired most of the time to retain the energy to have nemeses, especially nemeses who are women. Everyone honestly seems like they're trying their best to survive and make art within capitalism, and this is what patriarchy does—tries to pit women against one another, to compete for the very few slots of attention or recognition at the top. I still have a couple of male nemeses who are writers, as it feels healthy to have a nemesis, or, plural, nemeses, when writing, just as it's helpful to have an addressee. I realized today, because of some tabloid piece I was reading, that Amal Clooney and I are the same age, approximately. However, the Internet lists Amal Clooney as only forty, which is her age, as she was born in February of 1978. It's strange to realize once I reached forty how friends I thought were much older than I am are only a few years older, even though I thought I was much younger, or at least younger, than they are. It felt more pronounced when I was thirty-five, and they were, say, forty-one. But now that I'm forty, or, as the Internet has it, forty-one, and they are forty-six, it doesn't seem too large a difference. It seems I either have friends who are five years older than me or five years younger. I know few women who are exactly my age. The ones who are older now refer to "getting older" like we are in the same category. Some of them are entering or have entered menopause, and so that is a difference, as I am still, apparently, fertile, but who knows for how much longer. However, those who are younger, still firmly in their thirties, no doubt think that I'm much older than they are. The gap closes on one side but widens on the other. I have no doubt my male nemeses spend very little time thinking about this, how they are no longer considered young once they turn forty, and what that means in terms of how they are perceived as writers and as people, and this is one of the reasons why they stay my nemeses. Sometimes it surprises me, the ages of celebrities, in terms of my own perception of my age. I've been doing a lot of Internet searches on the ages of celebrities, because I've been wondering whether or not to try to have a second child, which I've spent far more time thinking about than I ever spent thinking about whether to have one child, which I never spent much time thinking about, having thought the matter was already decided until I found myself pregnant. There are many online slideshows about the ages of actresses in Hollywood. For instance, "Women who have had babies past 40." I look at those lists a lot. They are the same lists, but I keep on looking at them. Or, when I find out how old a female celebrity or artist is, if they have had children, I find out the age of their children and subtract. Amal and George Clooney's twins will turn one year old in two days, I discover. That means that Amal was thirty-nine when she had them, so she's not on any lists. If she has another child, which in this interview with *The Hollywood Reporter* she says is not happening, as she was already "old" when she had the twins, then she would be on some lists, for sure. It's strange that as I get older, celebrities get older as well. I never expected that to happen. I often look at these celebrities who are forty or over forty and wonder if that's what that age looks like on me. And yet these celebrities are extremely well preserved. So if anything, I probably look much worse. I think that Amal looks, obviously, amazing. But she seems older than me, despite looking so young and radiantly beautiful and well slept in photographs. I wonder if it's because she obviously has a career and incredible accomplishments. Whereas I often wonder what it is I have accomplished, not owning my own home, not being employed full-time anywhere, at forty. I mean, her twins are one, but she's already so slender and out of the house. She doesn't lie around on the couch writing little things in her notebook and eating bagels and cream cheese. Of course, she is probably more well rested. I imagine Amal and George Clooney have a nanny, maybe two nannies, despite how he talks in magazine profiles about diaper duty. I'm imagining George Clooney, who is fifty-seven, doesn't lie around all day either, worrying over his age. I bet when he found out he was having twins, he didn't google other dads having babies in their fifties. He still looks charming, and dapper, and like—like himself—but when did George Clooney get old? When I see him, grayer, older, I realize then—I too have gotten grayer and older. Every year, it seems, this is happening.

DOUBLE

The poet and I share the same birthday, although we are a decade apart, which is to say I am a decade older than him. When I found out that we had the same birthday, I thought that this must somehow explain the instant kinship I felt with him, also because we both came from lower-middle-class Catholic backgrounds, backgrounds we had somehow transcended, or wanted to transcend, by being writers. On my first birthday while living in this city, we decided to meet up. We ate salads at a vegetarian restaurant and then went to a bookstore where he bought me the hardback of Wittgenstein's *Philosophical Investigations*. I still read the poet's inscription every time I look at it. I often think about how Wittgenstein thought his book was a failure, but he thought he should publish it because he was worried about his students plagiarizing his ideas from his lectures before he published them. It was generous for the poet to buy me the book, which was expensive. He was effusive like that. Often he paid for our meals with a credit card that he then expensed as a business meeting for tax purposes. I have often found poets, especially the poets who live in this city, to be the most money-minded and hierarchical of writers, perhaps because they have to be. The poet was interested in knowing every famous writer possible to know, and he would often mention these friends to me. I don't know if that's why we became estranged, his nature I might describe as *arriviste*. I think it could have been something I said or did, or didn't say or do. My friendships with writers I've met in this city have often fallen apart, having begun too fast and having often felt transactional. Even though we are no longer friends, we still write to each other on or around our birthday. He often communicates with a flurry of emojis that can vibrate or send out confetti. One of the last times I saw the poet was at a dinner party at his apartment, where he sat me next to a magazine editor he was hoping would write a profile of him someday, which happened, I noticed with some bemusement, last year. At the party, he told the story of how he got into the private university that he attended, despite not excelling in school. His acceptance letter was written to his name and address, but referenced different information than what was provided in his application. He realized that another student, with his same name, which was not an uncommon name, was the one accepted. He went to the school anyhow, met well-connected people, became the assistant to a famous writer, and even became a fairly famous poet himself, as far as the limits of that go.

W. AT THE MOVIES

After one of his Cambridge lectures, the philosopher would need to go see a movie. He would sit in the front row and let it wash over him, "like a shower bath," to try to expunge the disgust he felt for himself. His favorite actresses were Carmen Miranda and Betty Hutton. In 1949, he traveled on the *Queen Mary* third class, to visit his friend and former student, Norman Malcolm, in Ithaca, New York. He wouldn't let his friend pick him up upon arrival in New York City. Perhaps, the philosopher wrote to him, I'll meet a beautiful girl on the boat who will help me, just like in the movies. He also joked that he hoped to be introduced to Betty Hutton. At that point he felt too anemic to practice philosophy anymore. He was diagnosed with prostate cancer after returning to England and died soon after. He didn't live to see the breakdown of his favorite star Betty Hutton, whose film career ended due to a contract dispute at Paramount in the early 1950s. Afterwards she worked in radio, in Las Vegas nightclubs, in television, and did a stint on Broadway. In the late '60s, when the actress was in her forties, her depression and addiction to various pills worsened, co-inciding with the collapse of her fourth marriage, bank-ruptcy, and the death of her mother in a house fire. She had a nervous breakdown and attempted suicide when she lost her singing voice a couple years later. Eventually she converted to Catholicism and worked as a cook and housekeeper at a rectory in Rhode Island. The philoso-pher didn't live to see her path converge with his. In the summer of 1920, he also had a breakdown and went to work at a monastery, as a gardener.

AUTHOR PHOTO, PART ONE

Roland Barthes is smoking a cigarette.
James Baldwin is smoking a cigarette.
Karl Ove Knausgaard is smoking a cigarette.
Clarice Lispector is smoking a cigarette.
Marguerite Duras is smoking a cigarette.
Susan Sontag is smoking a cigarette.
Alejandra Pizarnik is smoking a cigarette.
Paul Bowles is smoking a cigarette.
Jean Genet is smoking a cigarette.
Yukio Mishima is smoking a cigarette.
David Wojnarowicz is smoking a cigarette.
Ingeborg Bachmann is smoking a cigarette.
Roberto Bolaño is smoking a cigarette.
Samuel Beckett is smoking a cigarette.
Carson McCullers is smoking a cigarette.
Thomas Bernhard is eating an ice cream cone.

WITHDRAWN

I find myself often thinking of a writer I used to correspond with, who every decade publishes, or published, a slim, witty novel of language and ideas. When I first began writing in public, around when my own first slim novel came out, we would leave comments on each other's blog posts and then would continue the conversation in long email chains. But I haven't heard from her since I began publishing books on larger presses and moved to this city. This also coincided with the publication of her last novel, which she had worked on diligently for an entire decade, which, once published, was met mostly with silence. Although my move to the city had nothing to do with publishing, I was aware of an impression that I had suddenly become a writer of this city. By the time this writer and I had begun communicating she had withdrawn largely from her literary community, or communities, in despair over the hostility of what she would call the *poetics coteries*, and when we stopped communicating I got the impression she had decided to withdraw from her friendships with writers completely, or at least from me. Or, I wonder now if it was in fact I who withdrew from her? Our references to each other were not only of quotes from Foucault, Duras, or Blanchot, but also of film, like our longing for writing that was like the cinema of Wong Kar-wai. After a lengthy conversation about a theory of emotions in literature, both reading emotionally and emotional works, it turned out we both considered *Broadcast News* to be one of our favorite movies. It was one of the first movies that made me realize something mainstream could be art, she wrote me. Like Billy Wilder but in the '80s. I had written to her that I often wish I could be like Holly Hunter, allowing myself to voluptuously weep once a day, as if to clear the pressures from my life. She wrote me that sometimes when she feels like she is totally losing it she wishes she could channel that scene where Albert Brooks puts on a French or Spanish pop song and begins mouthing along expertly to the words. I knew exactly what scene she meant, as I thought about it often and have watched the clip online countless times since then. Albert Brooks on the couch mixing the margarita in the glass with his two fingers, singing along to Francis Cabrel, guzzling the drink with both hands, falling back into the couch with that loud gulping sigh at the end. He has just been rejected professionally and, he senses, romantically. There is something rapturous to the mania of that moment, of being alone at home drinking while everyone else is working on the breaking story he has been shut off from, abandoned in favor of the blond, dashing William Hurt character, the sinking further and further in, like an ecstatic acquiescence to failure.

GHOST

We wrote to each other worried that S. hadn't written any blog posts for a while or left comments on our blogs. We hoped she was okay. Her husband, a Latin American poet who since becoming her ex-husband has won a major award, had recently left a comment on my friend's also pseudonymous blog. This felt like some sort of rupture in the fabric of community and semiprivacy that we had created. Did S. tell her husband the public identity of our friend, whose one novel in the '90s is now considered an important work of New Narrative, in its meditation on identity, language, and friendship? Had our covers been blown? S.'s husband had never commented on his wife's own blog—we didn't even know if he read it. My friend wrote me that she felt that S. was leaving her messages in the night somehow, but I didn't know whether she meant actual messages, like emails, or somehow psychic messages. My friend responded politely, even cheerfully, to the husband, the Latin American poet, in the comments of her blog, although I knew this breach of security meant my friend would most likely disappear forever from the Internet, worried over others finding out her identity. It wasn't supposed to be about names and who knew whom, but conversations about literature. My friend wrote me that the husband leaving messages as opposed to our friend S. felt like a story in Bolaño's *The Return*. Later, after we had been out of contact for a while, I read the collection. For a while I thought she was referring to the title story of *The Return*, when the narrator dies on the floor of a Paris disco and finds out to his horror that the move into the afterlife is exactly like that scene with Patrick Swayze in *Ghost*, where he sees a diaphanous ghost version of himself floating above his dead body. The story later advances into a plot about necrophilia. I realized that this couldn't be the story my friend meant, but rather another story in Bolaño's *The Return*, but even reading through it now, I have no idea which one. What is wonderful about Bolaño, my friend wrote to me at the time of our correspondence, is that his main characters are poets and revolutionaries.

SECOND DOG

For a long time we wanted to get a second dog. Then we had a baby, and I had to give up this desire for a while. Now I might want a second child. I also still want a second dog. When I think about getting a second dog, I think about what we might name the dog. It's exciting that we won't have to disguise naming the dog after a writer or artist. Our dog is named Genet, and I fantasize about a little terrier named Violette Leduc, so if our Genet ignores her or humps her, I can pretend I'm enacting some literary gossip, as Violette Leduc always abjected herself to Genet in her desire for his friendship. With babies, there is more pressure to at least disguise one's pretensions. Our daughter is named after Leonora Carrington, but we call her Leo. On the playground she plays with a girl named Cy (after Cy Twombly), a Willa (after Willa Cather), and a Nico. There was a Joaquin today. There is an Emile (or

Emil)—we don't know whether if that's after Zola, or, what I originally thought, Cioran, although the name might have nothing to do with writing at all. I have no idea what we would name the second child. I scan my bookshelves and nothing feels right. Perhaps this is a sign we are not going to have a second child. I think it's more likely we will get a second dog.

JOHN WAYNE

On a recent Saturday I attended my four-year-old niece's birthday party up in Westchester, New York. The party was held at a gymnastics center in one of those half-occupied corporate campuses. The adults stood around watching small bodies bouncing up and down in anticipation while waiting in line to jump up and down on a trampoline. There was something exhausted to the way we all stood around in clumps, saying hello or making small talk, watching for the tiny bouncing body that was ours. The previous birthday parties I had attended of my sister's two daughters had been held in the backyard of my sister's house, as they were born at the beginning and then the end of the summer. The parties usually featured some entertainment—a clown, a balloon man, a puppeteer, a bouncy house, or some combination of these things—and beer, which was helpful so the adults could have something to hold in their hands. There was no beer at the gymnastics center, although when the immediate family went back to the house afterwards, my sister did offer me a beer, which I accepted, although I wasn't able to drink it, having forgot where I placed it, as can happen when one is around small children. My father and my aunt, his sister, were there, having driven in from the Chicago suburbs, as my father doesn't like to fly. My father tries never to miss one of his grandchildren's birthday parties. My aunt and father stood around at first, while on the bouncy mats at the gymnasium, making some small talk with the adults, and later ate their pizza speechlessly in what was known as the party room, where all of the four-year-olds played their toy kazoos at once. My father and aunt were likely exhausted from the travel, but also exhausted because they are old and in poor health. They were exhausted before all the standing. I observe on this trip that my father has gotten heavier and seems less mobile than before. When my father measures the distance between the last time he saw my one-and-a-half-year-old daughter, he observes that she's become more mobile even though it's only been a few months, and I observe he's become less mobile. My aunt, who I haven't seen since last summer, seems to have lost weight, although she is still not very mobile. They both seem gray and unhappy. A startle to realize that my aunt is only in her late sixties—not so old, I tell myself, but only because I myself have gotten older. My aunt is now a senior citizen, but she is still the baby of the family, and my father, being her last surviving sibling, takes it upon himself to try to look after her, as she in turn looks after him. In this way when together they resemble an old married couple, which I realize the adults in the room probably think, if they don't know my sister well, which most of them do not. Still, I am a kid to them, even though I am suddenly a middle-aged adult. On this visit, my father and I take my daughter to a playground near where I live. Over this trip—where I see them only twice as they are staying near my sister's, which we all prefer—both my aunt and my father tell me that they each bought a new television set. My father has now told me several times he bought a new television set, and each time I let him tell me again, as if for the first time. My father's new television set is much larger—seventy inches, he says, to which each time, whether over the phone or now in person, I attempt some sort of noise that seems appropriate to the amount of space his new television set takes up. However, I have no idea how many inches the television set that's been in his living room for the last decade was, and how it compares to the new one. His son, my brother, the computer science professor who lives in the Midwest and is far more dutiful than I, helped him install it, he tells me. He still has the same, much smaller second television set in the basement, or perhaps he moved the larger set upstairs downstairs, replacing the much smaller set, but he doesn't watch television down there anymore, he tells me. I have a new television set, he tells me, which I interpret as another way of saying: I am not going down the stairs anymore. Also, as we sit on the bench at the playground and watch my daughter go down a slide, he tells me, after much nudging as to the state of his health, that he's worried about not passing his night-vision driving test, so he's also saying: I got a new, larger screen so I can see better. On the television set he watches a different John Wayne Western every night. He has a collection of 250 Westerns, he tells me, which seems like an exaggeration, although likely not all are John Wayne movies. The Internet just told me that John Wayne made "at least 73 films." My father has mostly stopped reading—he is, or was, an avid reader of histories and biographies—but he still watches one Western a night. My father also tells me, again, that recently he also purchased a new, much larger fish tank. Although he doesn't wish to go on trips to Italy, or buy new clothes, even though all of his clothes are worn, he chooses to buy a new, much larger television set, and a new, much larger fish tank, all in the living room, where he spends the majority of his time. So he has two new, larger screens—on one he watches John Wayne, and the other, fish swimming by. Although my father has to stand to watch the fish, as he cannot reorganize the living room space, which has been the same configuration since my mother died fifteen years ago. She died in that living room, in a hospital bed facing the television set, which was not on, as my mother didn't like to watch TV, and by that time, she wouldn't have been able to see it or hear anything anyway. It would be nice, I tell my father, while sitting on the park bench, feeding my daughter some of her granola bar, if you could find a way to be able to sit on the couch and watch the fish swimming by, as opposed to standing over them, which doesn't seem relaxing at all. But while saying this, I also realize the problems he has getting up from a couch now, which I observed at my sister's house, so perhaps he'd rather stand while watching them. While at the birthday party I speak to my aunt much less, as she irritates me, mostly because of the tone in which she talks to me, and the way she calls me Katie instead of Kate, but she also tells me she got a new television set in her living room, the house my father and she were born in, where she lives now all by herself. She feels guilty, she tells me, throwing out a perfectly good television set, which also annoys me, my family's extreme thriftiness. I can picture them both in their own living rooms at night, sitting in each of their armchairs that have grown dingy and thin, with the impression of their bodies and past bodies. I do not know what my aunt is watching on the television set, but I know my father is watching a John Wayne film, one he has already seen many times before. I think there is something relaxing to my father about that repetition. He knows the story line, and the history has already happened. The last time I was home, or at my father's house, was two years ago, when I flew in to take my father to specialist appointments, as he had a health scare. I promised my father that that night we would watch one of his row of DVDs. I picked *The Man Who Shot Liberty Valance*, as it was directed by John Ford and stars Jimmy Stewart alongside John Wayne. I hoped it would be a Western that artfully commented on Westerns. Jimmy Stewart is my father's second favorite actor, after John Wayne, and I've always suspected this is because both of these actors were Reagan Republicans, like my father. Also the film stars Vera Miles, who my father and I both like, me for *Psycho*, and him for *The Searchers*. It was such a strange film, *The Man Who Shot Liberty Valance*. I'm still thinking about it. What was strangest to me is that Jimmy Stewart and John Wayne also played younger men, as the film flashed back twenty-five years, to their youthful idealism in a small frontier town. They were supposed to be very young in the flashback scenes, and probably in their forties in the present-day scenes, but both actors were quite obviously in their fifties. The film opens in the present day with a funeral for the John Wayne character, a rancher who is one of the last cowboys, who the Jimmy Stewart character, now a politician, insists can still wear his boots in the coffin. I think this was supposed to symbolize that the West, as they knew it, was also now dead. There was something so grating about John Wayne's voice, the way he kept calling the Jimmy Stewart character "Pilgrim," but I assume that what I found grating in tone my father felt soothing. I wonder if when we watched it together, in the basement of my father's house, I thought about my father, and his eventual funeral, especially since he was at the time very sick, but would then get better. While writing this I also remember a strange event that occurred while on the playground during my father's visit. While I helped my daughter around the jungle gym, teaching her how to go down a slide, a talkative five-year-old asked me if I was my daughter's grandmother or grandfather, which I had no idea how to react to, although my father laughed it off. How strange that she would think I was so much older than I obviously was. Then I realized, mathematically, I could have been her grandmother. It wasn't that she didn't understand my gender that bothered me, but that she assumed that I was old. But of course to her I was old, even if I could be made still to feel so young.

BECKETT IN SHORTS

Those photographs of Beckett strolling around the square in Tangier with his collared shirts and short-shorts that show off his tanned stork legs. How cheerful he looks. Smiling! In 1978 he was seventy-two years old. Beckett's plays are obsessed with age, like Krapp listening to his past monologues on an old tape recorder on his sixty-ninth birthday. It was on holiday in Morocco that Beckett found inspiration for the visual imagery for his short play "Not I." In a café he watched a woman waiting for her child to get off from school, which inspired the play's silent Auditor, clad in a djellaba, who makes isolated gestures of compassion as he or she observes words pouring out of the Mouth floating above the audience. To play the Mouth, Billie Whitelaw had to be strapped into a sort of vise, elevated eight feet above the stage, where she couldn't see or hear anything and so had to memorize the fourteen-minute monologue, which narrates with incredible speed the sad, lonely life of a woman about seventy: her early parental abandonment, her unspecified trauma, lying facedown in the grass, standing in line in a grocery store. The visual of the open mouth was inspired by Caravaggio's painting of the beheading of John the Baptist. Beckett preferred Billie Whitelaw's performance to Jessica Tandy's, who debuted the role in New York. Whitelaw, his favorite actress, knew how to make it mechanical, automatic, just like the voice in Krapp's tape recordings. The Auditor disappeared after the early performances. How many times I've watched the film version of Billie Whitelaw in "Not I" on YouTube. "It looks like a vulva!" Beckett exclaimed after seeing the close-up of her mouth on screen.

AND I

(after Borges)

The other day, I read a story in which I was a character, or at least the other "I" that has my name, who is an author, was a character. The story—or was it more of an essay?—was written by my friend M., who I actually wrote about in my last novel and, I suppose, am writing about in this story now. I think the "I" in the story—or was it an essay?—was less the friend who communicated with M. about our children, our writing processes, our various complaints, or the private matters of needing time, but the "I" she first met while reading my books. It was an unsettling experience, to be made a character in someone else's writing. I confess, I didn't like it. Although, more so, I didn't like that the other "I," the one who shared my name, was the character. It would have been better, I think, if I, the I who is I, were the character instead. It was a splitting feeling. I realize the author-I and the other-I are in some ways the same person, in that we both share a love of Roland Barthes, of famous hermits, and of slow film, but the author-I is interested in all of these things in a showy, off-putting way, as if to announce her interests to the world. I realize writing this that in reading M.'s story a third "I" emerged who shared our name, that of someone else's character.

My friend M. and I have a lot in common—I imagine she experiences a similar strangeness when she is written about in my work. We have often quoted to each other Foucault's line "I am no doubt not the only one who writes in order to have no face." The way Foucault says, "I am no doubt not the only one," is in fact a gesture of friendship.

Of the three "I's" that exist, I do not know which of us is writing this now.

AUTHOR PHOTO, PART TWO

After a haircut: "You look more like yourself again."
When asked to elaborate: "Well, more like *photographs*
of you."

SONTAG IN THE BEAR SUIT ONE

Susan Sontag follows you around in a bear suit, offering trenchant critique, but only you can see her, like an update of *Harvey*.

SONTAG IN THE BEAR SUIT TWO

. . . but how does she manage to still look so serious?

REFORMER

My Pilates instructor, Y., who I've been going to in order
to attempt to push my abdominal muscles back together
after delivering a nine-pound baby, is an interesting con-
versationalist. I think I might go to her simply to talk to
her, as I don't have any other friends in the neighborhood, though Y. and I are not really friends, the reality
is I pay her to stand over me and force me to execute
various small and slow movements with my legs, torso,
and abdomen, both on the mat and on various machines,
all while she tells me to get organized. Okay, now get
organized, she says to me, looking critically at my body,
before I am to begin a series of movements. She looks at
my soft middle and thinks of ways to correct it, and I,
in turn, attempt to do what she tells me, even though I
often complain, and try to get her to talk about her life,
which slows us down. She just got back from a medita-

tion retreat where she didn't speak for a week. She had a look on her face in our sessions afterwards, like it was disorienting to have to use her mouth again, to have to explain to an unfit person how to move her muscles in a specific way, as so much of Pilates is about very specific movements and routines, most of which I haven't learned yet, as I'm still a beginner, despite having gone to her for several months. Y. goes to see plays and dance often, and since I haven't figured out yet how to leave the house really, except for errands or to teach or for these sessions, I like to get her reviews, which are always negative, or at best indifferent. She often goes because a friend has a ticket. She just saw Misty Copeland perform with the American Ballet Theatre, which you could tell she found annoying, as the theater was crowded with celebrities, she said. Like what celebrities, I asked, as I was doing leg-work on the Reformer and she stood over me, pressing on the bandages on my feet, to keep me in the right position. I was breaking in a new set of summer clogs, and she kept on remarking on my bandages, that they looked like the color of skin in an Alex Katz painting. Later, she brought this up again. Oh, your Alex Katz Band-Aids. Oh, you know, she said, in that specific way of hers. Like, Marla Maples. I really enjoyed the way she said "Marla Maples," and also thought it was funny, her example of a celebrity in the audience. Maybe the tone of her voice and her example was a way to tell me that there were bad celebrities in the audience, annoying celebrities. Y. speaks with a slight Japanese accent, as she spent her adolescence in Japan, as she's Japanese, but also with a twang that I found deeply familiar when I met her. During our first session, we realized that she spent her childhood only a few miles away from where I grew up, in the nondescript strip mall landscape of the northwest suburbs of Chicago, before moving to Japan. When we discovered this, it made me then realize that I was drawn to her partially because of this, because of how she spoke. I never meet someone from there, she said to me, and I agreed it was unusual. If I was going to project, I would say perhaps we were both a little embarrassed, as this was not a glamorous place to be from, or to have lived, and I guess you'd only know this if you were from there. I asked her if she remembered going to the Pickwick, the dollar theater in Park Ridge, and she did, and I felt disoriented then, talking about this, there, with her, after all of this time, and I remembered then the floors of the theater, sticky with Coke, and when I was a senior in high school seeing that Meg Ryan movie there where she's drunk and hiding it while married to Andy Garcia, but one time gets so wasted that she crashes through the glass door to her shower, and has to go to rehab. I find Y. a pleasant mix of contradictions. She goes to silent retreats, but she is also a name-dropper. When I told her I was a writer, as I was lying down on the Reformer the first time, she said she wasn't a reader, but then asked me if I knew her really good friend who was a famous novelist. I didn't know him, but I knew who he was, as he had a recognizable name. I don't know if she was really good friends with him, or was friends with him, or just knew him, although also didn't know why she would lie. She also tells me the famous people she's met while being a fitness and health devotee in the city over the past two decades (she is a few years older than me). Like that Madonna took yoga with her in the '90s. The last session we had, as we were stretching out on the floor, she thought I had said "Kennedy" (I hadn't, I think I said the word "cocktail," but now I don't know why) and began telling me that she used to teach a couple Kennedys. I had no idea which Kennedys she meant, the lesser female Kennedy cousins, I suppose. It's so sad about them, Y. said to me. And I asked her what she meant, thinking she was referring to family tragedy. They have the most beautiful bodies, she said to me. But all the women in that family have that Kennedy face.

RIDER

A silhouette of a cowboy on his rearing horse revealing a partial photograph of a Natalie Wood press photo underneath (white opera glove, cleavage)—against a saturated red background, one of Sarah Charlesworth's red photographic collages. Something like a centaur or another hybrid creature. Natalie Wood before her mysterious death, drowned off the coast of Catalina Island in 1981 after going missing from the family yacht, *Splendour*. (That scene between Natalie Wood and Barbara Loden in 1961's *Splendor in the Grass*, the two mirroring each other. Barbara Loden as party girl Ginny Stamper, Warren Beatty's sister, who tries to get her to have a drink from the flask. Come here, Deanie-Girl, she says. Natalie Wood as Deanie looks by turns nervous and unsure, flattered and excited, by her attention.) In a 1961 profile, *Time* magazine wrote, "Natalie Wood has every reason to feel exhilarated . . . she is just about the raciest filly to come down the Hollywood sound track since Liz Taylor." She resembles Elizabeth Taylor here, *BUtterfield 8* Elizabeth Taylor. Most likely a publicity shot for 1962's *Gypsy*. On the boat too was her husband, Robert Wagner; her then costar, Christopher Walken; and the captain. Natalie Wood was afraid of dark water—had she really been swimming? The autopsy revealed bruises on her body and a significant amount of alcohol in her system. She was forty-three years old. Natalie Wood is missing for the majority of *The Searchers*. John Wayne searches for her, but the film isn't about her; it's about the searching. Is Sarah Charlesworth referencing John Ford's silhouettes in the film, like the woman's shadow at the opening blacked out before the expanse of the Monument Valley landscape? John Wayne spends five years searching for his niece, Debbie, kidnapped by the Comanche. John Wayne plays a former Confederate soldier who takes years to return home after the Civil War is over, then sets off for years to avenge his slain family, and then, once that happens, sets off again. There is such rage to his hatred of the Comanche. It's unclear whether John Ford and John Wayne are commenting on his character's extreme racism, how it isolates him. There is some distance there, but how far, it's hard to know. Time works strangely in the movie. Natalie Wood's kid sister plays Debbie at the beginning of the film—she's about eight. But by the time John Wayne finds her, now a bride of the chief, Scar, she seems about seventeen or eighteen years old, even though only five years are supposed to have elapsed. Natalie Wood is in the film for all of a few minutes, and has almost no lines. She's there to be swept up (swallowed up) by these men looming over her on their horses. It's my father's favorite film. When I watch the film, again, I think about my father, at night, watching the film. When I see John Wayne, that shot at the end, leaving his homestead after delivering Natalie Wood to what remains of her home, I think of my father's loneliness, watching Fox News, and then watching John Wayne, alone in his house. I was so bored when I watched this film when I was younger. But watching it now, I realize that beyond the cowboy rhetoric this film is mostly about wandering through empty landscapes, about duration and time passing, the way that John Wayne and his sidekick move slowly through snow, through water, through desert, through seasons. The artist Douglas Gordon remembers his parents showing him *The Searchers* while growing up in Scotland. He has said it was his first experience with boredom. His parents told him the film was about searching and waiting, searching and waiting, and that he'd understand it when he was older. In *5 Year Drive-By*, his installation in the California desert, he tried to stretch the narrative of *The Searchers* to its real-time duration, 113 minutes to five years. A second of film lasted approximately six hours. The installation lasted seven weeks. He didn't do the entire film.

Viewers thought they were watching a stationary shot, most likely of John Wayne's face, but they were seeing instead a sequence. "As I'm sitting there, I'm thinking this is the artist who stretches things," says an interviewer for *The Brooklyn Rail*. Gordon replies: "The elasticity of it is interesting."

PINK BUNNY EARS

I find myself thinking a lot lately about Ray Johnson. The constellations of famous figures and friends that he put into his collages. How in those early years, in the 1950s, he carried these collages in boxes and shared them with strangers, mailed them to friends. He burned them in Cy Twombly's fireplace, an act that John Baldessari mimicked with his paintings in *Cremation*. "Please send to Peter Hujar," he writes in his pink-highlightered script at the bottom of the collage I saw at the Matthew Marks Gallery last summer. A postcard of an older Sophia Loren in leopard print with horn-rimmed glasses swinging a small child with a man on the other side. Ray Johnson drew pink bunny ears on the child and collaged over the child's torso a photo of a nude man with his arms raised vertically, his hands obscured by a wooden crossbeam, mirroring the pose of the child and also suggesting a crucifixion. There are so many other crucifixions in collages in the show. It's too small for me to see if this one is a Hujar photograph. I kept on looking at it—there were so many layers to it. How Peter Hujar rejected fame like Ray Johnson. That story of Hujar being introduced to Cecil Beaton at a party: "I hear you are a very fine photographer," Cecil Beaton said to him. "I hear the same about you," Hujar said, and walked away. When Ray Johnson was mugged at knifepoint in lower Manhattan on the same day his friend Andy Warhol was shot by Valerie Solanas—June 3, 1968, two days before Bobby Kennedy was assassinated—he left the city and moved to a small white hermitage on Long Island, with a Joseph Cornell attic, as he described. Many of his correspondents became famous. He became more and more reclusive, keeping in touch through his mail art and on the phone. Eventually he stopped selling his work. And yet both Peter Hujar and Ray Johnson were obsessed with stars and fame, like Ray Johnson's series of collages addressed "Dear Marilyn Monroe." He saw patterns in everything, especially numbers. That Marilyn Monroe was born in 1926 and died in 1962. The number 13 was important. There are thirteen letters in the name Marianne Moore, with whom Johnson kept a correspondence (like Joseph Cornell) and devoted a series of collages to, using as a reoccurring image her tricorn hat. The number 13 plays a role in decoding the patterns behind his suicide, which everyone thought must be a final Ray Johnson performance. He was 67 (6+7=13), and it was on January 13, 1995. The room number at the motel he had checked into earlier, 247 (2+4+7=13). He was seen dressed in black and diving off a highway bridge in Sag Harbor, Long Island, and was last seen backstroking into the sea. Hundreds of collages were found arranged in his home. "I've got to tell you, it's like doing a gigantic puzzle," the Sag Harbor police chief is quoted in the *Times* obituary. I feel like when I'm writing these little pieces I'm making a daily collage. Please send this one to Ray Johnson.

BETTE DAVIS HORROR FILM

I hadn't seen T. in many years, so I was surprised when she wrote me that she was visiting the city and asked if we could meet for a drink. I didn't want to say no, but I wasn't exactly looking forward to it. We had met working at the bookstore together in London a decade earlier, and I had dedicated my first novel to her, mostly because she was one of the only ones who read my writing, having kept in touch as a pen pal over the years. I think when I became a published author the shift caused a strain between us. She was partially the inspiration for the doppelgänger friend in one of my novels. I borrowed some of her mannerisms for the character, especially the way that she would launch into monologues describing the plots of entire films. T.'s cinephilia was partial to art horror, like Alejandro Jodorowsky and Takashi Miike. She always had a love of the bodily and weird. Her mother was a doctor, and she told me how she remembered playing with bones from a human skeleton kept in a closet as a child. Perhaps it wasn't a surprise then that since we knew each other, T. had gone to school back home in Australia to become a nurse. She seemed almost embarrassed that that's what she did now, working as a geriatric nurse, emptying bedpans. I think she may have wanted to be a writer, or a filmmaker, or to work somehow in film, but that never happened. While she was in the city, she told me, she was seeing a festival of Bette Davis horror films. She began telling me about the one where Bette Davis plays identical twins, one kills the other, and then has to be tried for murdering her husband, a crime that her twin, who she killed, had committed. I hadn't seen it; the only Bette Davis horror film I had seen was *What Ever Happened to Baby Jane?*, which is the first of what Renata Adler called the "Terrifying Older Actress Filicidal Mummy genre," otherwise known, Wikipedia says, as psycho-biddy, or Grande Dame Guignol films. So few of the star system actresses resisted that final chapter in which they starred in horror films playing grotesques of their former selves. Vivien Leigh wouldn't do it. Tallulah Bankhead, Joan Crawford, Veronica Lake, Bette Davis did. Bizarre, looking it up, that Bette Davis was only fifty-four and Joan Crawford fifty-six at the time they made *What Ever Happened to Baby Jane?*. Isn't it?

CINEPHILE

She was obsessed with literature and film but couldn't seem to find a way to make a life out of it. For a while she worked as a travel agent to a London-based private military contractor during the Iraq War. Like the kind that operates black sites? I asked her. She had no idea and didn't seem concerned. It paid a salary and good benefits and she seemed comfortable. I suggested perhaps she go to school to become a film archivist, or to think about working for a film festival, but she either wasn't interested or didn't see that as being possible. Perhaps she always wanted security, although she didn't own her own place or buy expensive clothes. She spent all of her money on traveling to see films at international film festivals, and on DVDs and books. She also asked me to make her a list of books she should read. She read everything I suggested, like all the Dalkey Archive Press books, even though those were expensive to get abroad. When we saw each other, after all these years had passed, she only wanted to talk about what books I had read and what films I had seen. I asked her if she had seen Abbas Kiarostami's *Close-Up*, which was a film I thought about all the time. The cinephile in the film is such a fan of the Iranian filmmaker Mohsen Makhmalbaf that he impersonates him when he meets a somewhat wealthy family, which he then enlists to make a film, until he is ultimately tried for fraud. This was based on real-life events that happened in the late '80s in Tehran. When the filmmaker Kiarostami heard about the trial, he immediately began work on a documentary about the impersonating cinephile, and received permission to film his trial, and also got the cinephile/impersonator and the family to agree to play themselves and reenact the events. At the end of the film when the impersonator meets the real-life Makhmalbaf, they ride together on a motorcycle through the traffic of Tehran, with Kiarostami's film crew attempting to follow behind. There was something about this film that encapsulated for me this longing to be near art, that the impersonator and the family all feel, to be near the making of it, but how shut out they felt from the possibility that they could live the life of an artist. I thought about this film when talking to the cinephile. Had she watched it? Of course she had.

PATTY HEARST WINS THE
WESTMINSTER DOG SHOW

Such nice movement in the flowing coat of Rocket the Shih Tzu, the winning top toy dog, as she walks for the judges in the green-carpeted ring at the Westminster Kennel Club Dog Show, held annually at Madison Square Garden. Two years later Patty Hearst's French bulldogs (her usual breed) also won top prizes. The media made much of the famous image of the newspaper heiress as Tania, posed for a Symbionese Liberation Army photograph, wearing a beret and brandishing a gun, having been kidnapped from her Berkeley apartment when she was nineteen. When I first moved to this city I tried to write a Kathy Acker–like riff for a Rotterdam-based art journal about the grainy black-and-white surveillance footage of Tania holding up Hibernia Bank, about the split images of Patty and Tania, plagiarizing lines from her ghostwritten memoir, and collaging it with the diary entry of the character of Patty in Jonathan Franzen's *Freedom*, but my attempt wasn't very good. I think it was too obvious. There was nothing that made me happier than various plays on the headline "Patty Hearst Wins the Westminster Dog Show." It combines my two favorite things—small dogs and lives post-fame. "'People move on,' she said, smiling at Rocket." Patty Hearst has grown-up daughters and grandchildren now. She is in her sixties. Dogs are her present-tense now. I place the photograph of Rocket with her hair held up in that purple bow, that little upturned face, next to the AP photograph of Patty Hearst with her hair held back, wearing a prim dress, being led from a federal building in handcuffs, and there is something there, in both of their expressions. I guess it's true what they say.

DOGS IN FILM

I

The little Italian greyhound that is always held in *L'Avventura*.

II

That moment in *A Single Man* when Colin Firth smells the head of the smooth fox terrier, remembering the smell of his own dogs, when they were still alive.

III

The eleven-second cameo in *The Birds* when Tippi He-
dren, in blonde halo, stands in front of Davidson's Pet
Shop, and turns around to enter as Alfred Hitchcock ex-
its quickly with his two Sealyham terriers Geoffrey and
Stanley (Sarah stayed home). Hitchcock gave Tallulah
Bankhead a Sealyham as a gift for staying to film *Lifeboat*
despite the harsh conditions of the shoot, being soaked
constantly in water, contracting two cases of pneumonia.
She named the dog Hitchcock.

DOGS IN VIDEO

The way Joan Jonas uses her three dogs as a form of inspired accident, as they run into the frame or nudge her to play ball, in her video works. She drew her dogs' heads over and over. Like a sickness, she has said. In her 2014 video *Beautiful Dog* she attached a GoPro camera to her poodle Ozu's collar so we could see the world upside down through his back legs.

LA CHAMBRE

The poet and I teach similar material in our writing seminars at the college, although hers is bracketed as poetry and mine as nonfiction. We seem to be interested in the same artists at the same time. I don't think she likes this, the poet, although it doesn't bother me. There was that time we were both writing about Sarah Charlesworth's Stills series. And now I see on her syllabus that she is teaching Chantal Akerman's *La Chambre* (1972). I am teaching it as well. I like thinking about how slow Akerman's works are, how they are about time and endurance and how this can connect to writing, I say to the poet. Yes, that's what I'm thinking about as well, she says. It makes sense we are both thinking about Akerman, as she had just died the year before. Writing this, I rewatch *La Chambre* on YouTube. This is the first film that Akerman made when she came to New York in the 1970s. The film is ten minutes and twenty-five seconds, a moving still around a small apartment. The slow rotation of a red-back chair, a table with a breakfast scene, like a Vermeer still life, oranges, apples, cups of coffee, coffeepot, croissant, a pack of smokes, the morning light of the window, the kettle on the stove, the bureau, the bedside table with more fruit, the young director lying in a rumpled bed, more chairs, a desk, a sink, a door, and again, as time moves throughout the day, various positions of Akerman in bed, sitting up, etc. When Barbara Loden saw Warhol's '60s films, like *Sleep*, which is of his lover John Giorno sleeping, or *Empire*, or I think it was *Chelsea Girls*, she said that she realized that a film could be boring. How Warhol purposefully slowed down the view of the Empire State Building in *Empire* to eight hours and five minutes. That film is an act of duration, of us watching time passing. I remember sitting through all three hours and forty-five minutes of Chantal Akerman's *Jeanne Dielman, 23, quai du Commerce, 1080 Bruxelles*, at the movie theater in Chicago, and again in London. As I spoke to the poet, I was sitting on a couch in my small temporary office they gave me for the semester, the office of a poet laureate on sabbatical. I was in my third trimester of pregnancy. How slow and fast time passed then and now. All day I stayed there, on that couch, meeting students, my feet up. I still remember—the bookshelves of that office, the large Rilke section, the many boxes on the floor, the empty laundry detergent containers under the desk, that phone that never worked, that printer that never worked, the fan.

GERTRUDE STEIN, ABOUT 3 PM
ON A SATURDAY

(after Anne Carson)

I will come with you to the party, I said, if I can be someone other than my name. If I can be a person who is not
my name, then I will come with you to the party.

NEW YORK

"Who does your foreign rights?" asked the philosopher, when I tried to speak to him about Wittgenstein.

PLAGIARISM

For a long time I worked on an essay about a fairly obscure American film made in the seventies by an actress, the only film she directed, that she starred in herself, an essay that I published in a small journal and thought perhaps I would turn into a book. For a couple of years it was all I worked on, slowly, as slow as the film itself. After the essay came out in the journal, I discovered a book in French that was about this same film and actress-director. It was written at approximately the same time as I had written my essay. This book won a significant literary prize in France and loving, critical attention for its English translation. I'm not saying it was the exact same text—her small, lyric monograph and my novella-length essay. For one, her book was more conceptually focused, while my essay drifted too much and was too much about me. Still, the similarities were uncanny. Had

I unintentionally plagiarized her, or had she unintentionally plagiarized me? The whole situation reminded me of that anecdote of Salvador Dalí throwing a fit when in the audience for the screening of Joseph Cornell's 1936 film *Rose Hobart*, which intercut the actress Rose Hobart's scenes in *East of Borneo* with shots from a documentary about an eclipse, projected through blue glass and scored by a record of Nestor Amaral's *Holiday in Brazil* that Cornell found in a junk shop. Knocking over the projector, Dalí accused Cornell of stealing the idea from his dreams. In a way, what the French writer and I were both doing was like Cornell's film—an homage to our actress, slowed down to the speed of a silent film. Still I see the book in bookstores, the cover with an illustrated still of the actress-director's face, and I feel that it is . . . not quite mocking me, you understand, but reminding me of something.

DREAM

I had a dream about M. last night. We saw each other in a large crowd. Then, the crowd thinned, and I became aware that M. was going to perform a couples dance with a man whose face I never saw and whose body I was even less aware of. It wasn't a competition but a performance. Her dancing partner flew her in the air. At some point she stood on top of a horse. It was not a surprise to me how good she was. M. is good at everything, I remember thinking in my dream. Afterwards, we found each other in the crowd, and were happy to see each other. You could really be a dancer, I said to her then. She was humble, as M. usually is. She was never good enough to go pro, she said, so she just does it for fun. I woke up in a panic, realizing I was expected to now be a professional writer. And I wasn't good enough. Or, I explained to M. over email, it wasn't what I wanted. If I could only write throughout my entire life with the electricity of the amateur.

INTRODUCTIONS TO
B. INGRID OLSON

BODY PARSED, THREE ROOMS

To write an introduction is to double oneself. Is to fold one's thoughts into another. To fold one's body into another body. To fold one's text into another text. What is my body and what is your body. What is my text and what is your text. What is my space and what is your space. We have to remove our limbs in order to fit inside this book. How to write an introduction for a book that will be destroyed after a certain period of time. Only those who are in the dark room can read it. Is this utopian, I wonder. I stay inside a dark room and write. Time has a different insistency now.

I read Elizabeth Grosz's *Architecture from the Outside*. I copy half of it down in my notebook, and then can't read my handwriting. From her introduction: "One cannot be outside everything, always outside: to be outside something is always to be inside something else." I like thinking about this but don't really know what this means. I write this out on a pad of paper; my hand hurts. I am in the room reading. I am on the couch. I type this out on my computer, and my laptop becomes part of my body. I am inside this book; I am inside this room; I am inside this body; I am outside this book; I am outside this room; I am outside this body. In my notebook I write this down again, to try to understand it: "One cannot be outside everything, always outside: to be outside something is always to be inside something else."

I ask the man in the room with me what I should write about. I ask, Do you remember when I spoke about this book, the one that had open windows and doors? Does it have open windows or doors, or does it have no windows or doors? I ask, Do you remember when I was inside of it, and I could not go outside of it, the book became my body, or was my body always a book? While waiting to write my notes on this book, I drink a green smoothie that he made for me. I name a future and imaginary child. I become the couch, scattered with books and notebooks. I look at boots online for my feet. I write three emails. I look at a photograph on my phone of a pregnant body. I google "Why does my baby have red cheeks?" I receive a package in the mail. I write this introduction while very full, and crouched over a pillow on the couch, and in another position, my legs in the air. I write this introduction while wearing leggings and an open robe, my breasts accessible. I write this introduction while wearing the same white set of overalls with coffee stains for four days. My body is a sentence. These gestures are ellipses.

Time has passed. It's been years. I have been asked to add a note to the second edition. My feelings about the book remain the same.

FOREHEAD AND BRAIN

I realized I was extremely miserable when I wrote the previous introduction. Now I am extremely happy. Or perhaps I was happy the entire time. I read a paragraph and then have to rest. I lie down on the sofa. I lay the book down. I lay myself down because I am now the book. I write a sentence and then have to check my email. After I write I am hollowed out. Do I even have a brain. I put the book up to my forehead and lay it on my brain. I put the book on my crotch and take a photograph. I wonder whether the book is a container, and what it is a container for. Perhaps it is a container for thoughts. Perhaps it is a container for language. Perhaps it is a container for memory. It is something like a brain. Is the mind a room. I spend time looking at images of the illustrations of the brain from Vesalius's *The Fabric of the Human Body*. I want to write about the Dark Room of This Book, furnished with a stretched cloth. A frame with cloth stretched over it is a painting. A frame with cloth stretched over it is a body. A frame with a cloth stretched over it is a window or a table. The body is a house. Vesalius was one of the first to dissect human beings in a surgical theater, not just animals as before, because of religion. He dissected the brains of convicts, most likely. He thought there was just fluid in the ventricles, not the soul like everyone else. Medical illustrations want to make the body an open window so we can see the structures within. What is a skull but a vitrine for the brain. What occupies the theater of the forehead is the front matter, the dura, the folds. Now we know something of what the cerebral cortex stores, in future mappings of the frontal lobes: movement, speech, memory, intelligence. I look at an illustration of Vesalius's horizontal dissection of the brain. The strange illustration of the man with the beard and nose, his head hollowed, like he is awake or surprised.

UNHINGE NAME TURNS MEMBRANE, BODY TO COME

When the question is raised of writing an introduction, one thinks that the books that need introductions are those that are opaque, and are thus impertinent to introduce. This is supposed to be an entrance or window. I wanted to have four cells on this page. Four cells would be a grid or window. The book is a dark room entitled *New Essays*. I wanted this writing to be all interior. The self must be more than what is inside and outside. What is not the self.

When writing *The Passion According to G.H.*, Clarice Lispector was going through difficulties in her family life, but the work eludes the autobiographical. It is only of a faceless woman alone in the room. She is frustrated by this "room." What can contain her. What is "narrative." What is "I." What is a "book." Who is to say. The room is unstable and becomes the narrator. "Before I entered the room, what was I?" G.H. asks. "I was what others had always seen me be, and that was the way I knew myself." When she enters her maid's room, she observes that the room is the portrait of an empty stomach. She enters into a dialogue with a cockroach that she decapitates with a door, then ultimately ingests its oozing entrails. One must ideally stand up when reading this. A text must be vertical and should be ingested within the body.

Over the period of hours during which I have written this introduction, I have lost my body, my human frame. Franz Kafka wrote his story "The Judgment" in one sitting from September 22 through September 23, 1912, from 10 PM to 6 AM. He writes in his diary that his leg grew so stiff from sitting over that eight-hour period that he had to physically pull them out from under the desk, like he had been cut in two. He felt, he wrote, such a fearful joy like the language came out of him so freely, like he was advancing over water, like he was not even a body. The story "The Judgment" takes place mostly in two separate rooms, the father is in bed, and the son is at his desk, and he goes back and forth, and they flow into each other.

I go back to my book. The psychotic person has their boundaries collapsed, and cannot distinguish between outside and inside, self and other. I have read this quoted in another introduction, because it is not likely you have read it, as the book is out of print. When Shulamith Firestone was found dead in her fifth-floor walk-up in the East Village, the authorities thought she might have been dead for some time, but her family did not permit an autopsy. She was thought to have a version of Capgras delusion, where one fears that loved ones are actually doubles, wearing masks of the formers' faces. When I first moved to New York City, I would walk to her apartment and stand outside, looking through the window, and would stay there for some time.

HEAD, HOUSE, LIGHT

Can a text be a house. Can a paragraph be a room. Can a sentence be a window. Wittgenstein's sister Gretl thought helping to design her large city house in Vienna would be a good activity for her brother the philosopher. Wittgenstein was still recovering from the war, and, he thought, philosophy. He was working as an assistant gardener at a monastery outside the city, and was mulling one of two possibilities for the future: either becoming a monk or committing suicide. He was in a form of exile, owing to what has been referred to as the Haidbauer incident, when working as an elementary schoolteacher at a village school in rural Austria, he hit an eleven-year-old boy, one Josef Haidbauer, so hard on the head during class that the boy collapsed and fell unconscious. There was a hearing, in which the judge requested a psychiatric examination—Wittgenstein fled, although he returned a decade later to apologize to the students, who were now older. Except for hitting the slower students, Wittgenstein was a wonderful teacher: he designed buildings and steamships with them, dissected animals, took long treks in the woods and identified plants, took the train to Vienna and discussed the various architecture of the buildings there. Even though he was a steel heir, he had given his fortune away, and slept in the kitchen, eating only oatmeal out of a pot he never cleaned. Of course, his family was concerned. There is a letter from his brother

Paul, the one-armed pianist, to one of Wittgenstein's friends, worried that his brother was not eating correctly for his colitis. He was supposed to only assist the architect, a student of Adolf Loos, on the design of the house, one of those cold modernist constructions of three white cubes. He was put in charge of the interiors: windows, doors, doorknobs, and radiators. As befitting the fastidious philosopher who once studied aeronautical engineering, he became absorbed in the project and completely took over, even moving into the small architect's office to live there full-time. He had to design the door handles himself, which took him a year. The heights for the door handles were minutely designed according to door type. It took another year to design the radiators. Each of the large vertical windows was covered with a metal screen, moved by a pulley system Wittgenstein designed. He insisted that everything be built according to exact proportions—including having the ceiling raised by thirty millimeters. He even wanted to make his own version of a head that he had disliked in one of the sculptures that were commissioned for the entranceway—his sister placed the plaster cast of the head he designed in the house. Of course, upon its completion, she didn't want to live there, and eventually the house was sold to the Bulgarian embassy. After finishing the house three years later, he returned to Cambridge and philosophy, wanting to work now on visual space. In his later *Philosophical Investigations*, he imagined thought as taking place in a room. "A person caught in a philosophical confusion is like a man in a room who wants to get out but doesn't know how." Wittgenstein himself liked to think in spartan surroundings—sometimes a chair in a room was all that he needed.

ON THE PUPPET THEATER

For a long time I was interested in puppets. This is what I studied in graduate school for the one year, performance theory, with a specialty in puppets. There was a story or essay, whatever it was, I read from that time, Kleist's "On the Puppet Theater," that he published in a Berlin newspaper in 1810. In this piece of writing, which is a dialogue of sorts, the narrator converses with a friend who is a dancer, about why he's so often in attendance at marionette performances in the town square. The dancer friend replies with a reverie about the graceful-ness of puppets, because of their mechanical nature. It is a mysterious piece of writing, something like a speculative essay. The conversation feels stilted, like the speakers are puppets and the writer is pulling their strings, making them walk and talk. It's always stayed with me. There was a time, after school, when I tried to apprentice with a local puppet theater. I didn't last long. I realized that to be a puppeteer I had to be good with a hammer, with making things, and I instead wanted to dreamily play with dolls, as I played with dolls until a very late age. I imagined being a puppeteer like something out of *The Double Life of Veronique*. After my mother died, so around this same period, I actually fell in love with a puppeteer. He was a Buddhist who had studied critical theory at Berkeley, and worked out at the same gym as Kathy Acker in San Francisco, or so he said. We would take long walks together and debate secular death, whether there was a God or an afterlife. He was a good deal older than me, deeply handsome, and very close to his parents. We waited a long time to have sex, because of his enforced celibacy due to a sex addiction, and when we did, he was often impotent. His last love was from a decade ago and was now an actress on an HBO TV show. I have a memory of us lying together, sexless, while Godard's *Breathless* played on a small TV screen at the foot of the bed, which even at the time I found somewhat ironic, or meaningful. He was a kind man who sat at my grandmother's dining room table and talked about people in the old neighborhood. He broke up with me because he thought I was too mean, or too young. I wish we had stayed in touch. He must be much older now. When I first moved here and saw the exhibit of Greer Lankton's puppets at Participant Inc, I thought of him. I had only known Greer Lankton before because of Peter

Hujar's black-and-white photographs of her, her graceful porcelain body, and also Nan Goldin's vibrant punk wedding photos. Greer Lankton grew up in Flint, Michigan, and began making dolls as an escape from bullying as a child, tormented by her gender. She died in Chicago of an overdose. I took so many photographs of her puppets at the show, her beautiful and grotesque dolls, of her Diana Vreeland, Candy Darling, Jackie O., these heroine shrines of a stylized femininity. I felt so alive being there.

SHORTS

There was the one who wore shorts every day, even in the winter. I wanted to know why. We hung out at the same bar. I found him charismatic, an intensity like he was from a different planet. He was tall with a bird face and sand-colored features. He had the same name as everyone else. I had heard, from his bandmate, that besides being a brilliant guitarist, he was also a writer, and had actually published a novel. It didn't seem like that could be true—that someone could publish a novel. Or maybe it was just stories, that he had published stories, or maybe he had just written a novel or stories. Maybe it surprised me because he didn't speak very much, but that's probably because he was on heroin. Everyone in his band, which was revered in that city, was from the same dingy suburban kind of town that I was from. One night, he followed me into the bathroom of the bar and

I let him, and we stood there, swaying at each other. After the bar closed, we talked like crazy people in the street. He would say something to me, quite close to my face, and then I would say something in response, and then he would say something, maybe grabbing my arm in protest, and I would say something, shaking my arm away, and it might seem like we were fighting or in some screwball comedy, but what he said did not correspond to what I replied. And so on. At one point he lunged at me and kissed me and our faces knocked together. Or did he cup my face with his large dry hands? We were standing by a stop sign. He took me home, to a tiny room with no bed in a larger apartment that at least one other girl occupied whom I remember meeting embarrassed around the kitchen island, which was right outside of his room, which was really a mostly empty room. Where do you sleep? I asked. He smiled again, in that eerie way. I think he just kind of collapsed on the floor and that's where he slept. I found myself being seduced by him still, despite him not having a bed. He showed me a picture of his ex-girlfriend who had just broken up with him. In the photograph she was completely naked. He didn't respond when I asked him things he didn't want to answer. Then he showed me some anal beads that were on his floor. He was laughing when he picked them up and showed them to me. What I wish I had asked, then, was whether these were clean anal beads or anal beads that he had recently used and then, removing them, threw them on the floor, or whether these were anal beads he had used with his ex or someone else, or anal beads he used on himself. We spent the night together. I mean, I think we spent the night together, but I don't know where we slept. We wrestled with our clothes on over his laundry for a while. He was a good kisser; his tongue was surprisingly agile and yet tender. For multiple reasons, penetration or removing our clothes seemed unlikely. By the end of our brief encounter, I still did not know why he wore shorts all the time, yet I felt sufficiently appeased in my curiosity. I began to dislike the way he and his friend, the lead singer, laughed at me. He would call me at home from the bar's pay phone or wherever he was on tour with his band and say my full name in that weird laughing drawl, then hang up. Since then, the lead singer of his band has become a successful novelist, or at least a published novelist. He's seen as a reclusive sort of underground artist in that city. The last time I was home was three years ago, and I went to a reading at a bar with S. The lead singer went up to me and began talking to me, as if he knew me, as if we were old friends or at least acquaintances. I wanted to say to him, You don't know me, the published writer, you knew that waitress you talked down to fifteen years ago, but I didn't say anything. I have tried to look up the boy in shorts to see what he's up to. He's still in the same band or set of bands. His Wikipedia page is only in German.

AUTOFELLATIO

The boy on the fire escape at the party told me of his manuscript that opened with an act of autofellatio. David loved it, he said to me, and even though I knew no real writers at the time, I still knew which David he meant. We made out a little, on the fire escape, even though he profoundly irritated me. I wonder if he wrote better than he kissed. I wonder if he ever published his novel.

REPLIES TO
MY MALE GRADUATE STUDENT

No, I still have not seen that documentary on Susan Sontag.

Thank you for noting the correct pronunciation of "Wittgenstein."

ANDREA DWORKIN!

You hear that a renowned biographer of women writers, a man, is writing an essay on the question of "female beauty" and genius. You hear this from your friend, a renowned novelist. Your friend tells you the biographer's working thesis is that women geniuses (writers and artists) are often described by their contemporaries as beautiful, even if we might think of their photographs as homely. So perhaps beauty is also the power or quality of mind, your friend writes you, or so this renowned biographer, a man, theorizes. You fire off a series of emails to your friend. You actively dislike, you write, the emphasis on a woman writer's appearance in conversations about her work. You are tired of reading that quote that Clarice Lispector looked like Marlene Dietrich and wrote like Virginia Woolf. This is distinct from acknowledging that Lispector's work is so much about vanity and the longing for beauty, ugly Macabea who wants to be Marilyn Monroe. And also, you write, about decreation, the desire to transcend beyond a face or the limits of a body. Sontag partially became Sontag because everyone took her photograph, yes, but the essays have nothing to do with her face. And are we talking about these writers' youth? Or when some of them created their greatest works, once they were older, when their work can often be about exploring this gap? The narrator in Duras's *The Lover* elegizing her face when young, how this face hasn't collapsed, has kept its contours, but still it is a face laid waste. And what about, you write your friend, Carson McCullers! (That photograph of the hunched-over McCullers having lunch with her friend Marilyn Monroe.) No one considered Simone Weil beautiful! Flannery O'Connor! Edith Wharton! Gertrude Stein! Violette Leduc was famous for her ugliness! Later in the day, one email, all caps—ANDREA DWORKIN!

Of course you realize later that this renowned biographer would most likely not think of Andrea Dworkin as a genius. Andrea Dworkin in her overalls. And yet the brilliance and intensity (even wrongness) of *Intercourse*. He wouldn't see it.

BURNED

"With my burnt hand I write about the nature of fire."
This is a line in Ingeborg Bachmann's *Malina*, often at-
tributed to Bachmann, although Bachmann is repeating
a line from a letter written by Gustave Flaubert. I am
collecting the slender obituaries in fiction of "the most
intelligent and famous female poet that our country
has produced in the past century," as writes her friend
Thomas Bernhard. Ingeborg Bachmann died at the age
of forty-seven in a hospital in Rome three weeks after
being badly burned in her bathtub, by a fire started from
a cigarette she didn't extinguish, having fallen asleep after taking what had become a regular diet of pills. The
circumstances remain mysterious. She was one of the
only people who seemed to like Bernhard as a person.
His grief spiky and clear in his brief story of her death
in *The Voice Imitator*, a death that he sees as some form of

suicide, a result of banishment, persecution, and exile, from not only her native Austria but also the jealousy of female rivals. A self-immolation. In *Malina* the narrator burns scraps of paper at night, as a way to light her cigarettes, the last cigarette, now another. This was the only novel that was finished in her *Todesarten* series, her Death Styles. Fleur Jaeggy mourns her friend in her brief story that recollects a memory of trying to speak with her of growing old together, but how old age seemed impossible for Ingeborg, a horror. The imaginary room of their old age furnished with blond Biedermeier. Jaeggy ends the story with years passing by in a sentence, then how she visited her friend every day in the burn unit at Sant'Eugenio. The story is entitled "The Aseptic Room." How a memory can feel like that. But is it ever a room free from contamination? Seven years earlier, in 1966, Clarice Lispector, another literary genius of the twentieth century, also famed for her glamour, almost died by taking a sleeping pill and falling asleep with an unextinguished cigarette, setting fire to her three-bedroom apartment in Rio de Janeiro. She was forty-six. Ingeborg was forty-seven. My friend M. who is that age, and a brilliant writer, writes to me today that she is reading a biography of Rainer Maria Rilke. She is getting to the part where he's dying, at the age she is now. When she turned that age, she wrote me, I am now the age of Max Ernst when he met Leonora Carrington, I am creepy-old-man age! Also the age of female geniuses setting themselves on fire, I could add, but don't. We are talking about other things. That night Clarice Lispector woke up to flames, and badly burned her entire body attempting to put out the fire with her own hands, in order to save her papers. Everything was lost. Her son Paulo dragged her out. Her nylon nightgown melted to her body. The bloody footprints across the carpeting. Her right hand, her writing hand, was completely disfigured. She spent the next three months in a hospital recovering, in terrible pain. She could eventually type with her hand again, although it resembled, her biographer writes, a blackened claw. Thankfully, her biographer writes, her face was not burned. Although this was the age her beauty left her entirely, he writes, the age of forty-six, her weight gain from her convalescence, although she was still striking, her famous beauty had now left her. She struggled with this, he writes. She had to remake herself completely; from this person who was Clarice Lispector, this name, she had to become someone else entirely. As I am writing this, I am thinking of how Susan Sontag's young son would stand by her desk as she wrote, lighting cigarette after cigarette.

SONTAG IN THE BEAR SUIT THREE

The photograph was taken by her partner Annie Leibovitz in Paris on New Year's Eve 2001. From *On Photography*: "All photographs are *memento mori*. To take a photograph is to participate in another person's (or thing's) mortality, vulnerability, mutability." She was to die three years later.

WE

We are skeptical of this writer if she gets too much attention—if her book got this much attention, there's a reason to be skeptical, we decide. However, we try not to be skeptical of our friends and their books. We are happy for their attention, and miffed if they do not get enough attention, like this other writer, why does she get so much attention, versus our friend, also a very good writer? However, if this other writer becomes our friend or friendly, or gracious about our writing, or our friends' writing, our skepticism can subside and we will try to read her book without judgment. Also, if some time has passed, and there is less attention, then it is possible to read her book without judgment. Sometimes then we decide it's very good, yes, worthy of all that attention, which we would have been unable to decide initially. And when the writer is dead we are even less skeptical. We are always like this—why? And all the others like this with us, inverse of our attention to theirs, etc. This is called "community."

PINK BEAR

I wrote a passage about the pink bear in the novel, but I found myself editing it out. In one of the first summers that I moved to this street, I saw a very large stuffed pink bear resting against a tree. The pink bear was as large as a full-sized person, or at least a short, full-sized person, but larger than a small child. The kind of sawdust-stuffed bear won at a carnival. It was slumped against the tree, in a posture that I saw as tender, in a way. It was like the bear was drunk, and someone had positioned it against the tree so that the bear wouldn't lose its balance and could sleep it off. I immediately took a photograph on my phone of the pink bear, and John, later, told me that he took a photograph of the pink bear as well. The fact that the pink bear was leaning against the tree on the sidewalk meant someone was throwing it out, but had enough care for the bear to lean it against a tree. The hope, by placing the pink bear against the tree, on or near the curb, was that someone could find it and take it home, like out of a children's book. My daughter has a children's book just like this. A girl finds a stuffed bear, slightly used, and takes it home to be her friend. My daughter loves this book. She likes it to be read to her every night. When I first encountered the pink bear, and then wrote about it, first in my notebook and later in a novel, my daughter didn't yet exist, and wouldn't, for a couple of years. Now, my daughter exists, although I'm not sure the pink bear exists, except in my memory, and how I've written about it, and how I am writing about it here. Although if the pink bear doesn't exist, where did it go? Perhaps no one picked it up—it was very large, it would be cumbersome to walk with down the street, and who wants a gigantic, cheaply made, slightly used pink bear? My daughter's grandparents sent her a very large, but still child-sized, stuffed bear that was also cheaply made, and it is difficult to store in our apartment. At first we tried hiding the bear, in closets, but my daughter always knew to look for it. There was something so wonderful to her about hugging a stuffed animal larger than herself, toppling it over. I wonder, what it would have been like if I had hugged the pink bear that I saw on the street, if I would have felt gently embraced and small in its gigantic arms. We finally got a container to hold my daughter's three other small stuffed animals, but mainly it's a container for her bear, to keep it out of our sight. The container cost more than all of the stuffed animals it holds. In one moment of trying to come up with a new game I dressed this bear in some of my daughter's old clothes while she watched, delighted, so now it wears an old sun hat falling off its head, and on one leg a small bathing suit from when she was a smaller baby, and an unbuttoned dress. When I originally wrote about the pink bear, writing about it reminded me that my mother would sew a birthday Care Bear every time I was invited to a child's birthday party. The birthday Care Bear was called Birthday Bear and had a pink cupcake with one candle on its white belly. All the Care Bears had names like this, Cheer Bear, Bedtime Bear, Friend Bear, Good Luck Bear, Funshine Bear, Grumpy Bear, Wish Bear, Love-a-Lot Bear, etc., and of course Birthday Bear. I didn't remember this until I just looked it up online, and now I remember it, vaguely. When I was younger, the Care Bears were really popular—there was a cartoon television show. Writing about the pink bear triggered this memory of the Birthday Bear. I realized the pathos of this as a repeat birthday present, something I didn't realize as a child. My mother getting out her heavy rose-colored sewing machine, and making a Care Bear from a pattern. A Care Bear that was a counterfeit Care Bear, and since she made a copy for each birthday party, children were receiving a copy of a copy of a Care Bear (itself a mass-produced doll), which must have not been received with as much pleasure as a Care Bear that was store-bought. With this memory, there's the pathos of three figures. The pathos of the thrifty mother, who must have spent hours stitching together the Birthday Bear, hours I never thanked her for or appreciated, as a way to budget presents for what must have been a stream of suburban children's birthday parties. There's the child (that's me) who has to bring this counterfeit Care Bear to the parties, and balance it on top of all of the wrapped, store-bought presents on the table. Then there is the child receiving the present, and forced to write a thank-you card and feign delight, which he or she did or did not do. Although I did not go to grade school with children whose parents had much money, so maybe they were happy with the gift. Maybe they didn't know the difference between a real and a counterfeit Care Bear. A stuffed bear is, after all, a stuffed bear. Perhaps I can only grasp the pathos of this from a distance of thirty to thirty-five years (as the Care Bears were created in 1981, the Internet tells me). Although, when I look at images of these sewing pattern Birthday Bears on eBay, I see that they really don't look at all like a stuffed bear, more like a stuffed pillow. I wonder what happened to all of these Birthday Bears. Or the gigantic pink bear from a couple of summers ago, and its gigantic pink siblings echoed across the city. Do any of them exist as friends in someone's room? Are there landfills occupied with cheap and counterfeit bears, piled high with their loneliness?

TALLULAH BANKHEAD

On a recent visit, while watching my young daughter play, my father at one point referred to her as Tallulah Bankhead. I'm not sure exactly why. Often I don't laugh at my father's jokes, but I found this funny, to call my baby Tallulah Bankhead. At the time my father didn't explain it, and he didn't wait around for the punch line to reveal itself, probably because he felt no one else would get the joke, but as I sit here thinking about it, I realize it's perhaps that Tallulah Bankhead—the actress—was famous for her "difficult" behavior, so an apt nickname for a toddler. It's possible in that moment my daughter was getting frustrated because she wanted to play with the ball being thrown to the dog, and was crabby because she had a molar coming in. I spend time getting lost on Tallulah Bankhead's Wikipedia page, which is twenty-two pages long (I printed it out). I watch the clip where she is on

The Lucy-Desi Comedy Hour, in the episode entitled "The Celebrity Next Door," a role originally slated for Bette Davis, before she cracked a vertebra. Bankhead, cigarette in hand, comes off as a Bette Davis replacement, as she sits on the couch in her black lace off-the-shoulder gown that matches Ball's lace dress. Her gestures and drawl, a mixture of stage British and Alabama, are almost too broad for television. Apparently she arrived drunk to rehearsals, to the frustration of Ball and Arnaz. There is a scene at dinner where for some reason Vivian Vance is waiting on them, in a maid's costume, and tells Tallulah Bankhead that she is such a fan as she lists her stage and film accomplishments, and Lucy tells her not to bore Ms. Bankhead. "I will tell you when I'm bored," Tallulah Bankhead then says, in that Tallulah Bankhead way. Later, Lucy will apologize for the "help," and say how old her maid is getting, the joke being that Vivian Vance, who is on the other side of the door, listening and reacting in comic disbelief, was actually only two years older than Lucille Ball. I had forgotten that Tallulah Bankhead was up for the role of Scarlett O'Hara, which would have been a revival of her career in Hollywood after a string of flops, but David O. Selznick thought she was too old at thirty-six to start out at sixteen and age more than a decade. Tennessee Williams was frustrated with her portrayal of Blanche DuBois in the 1956 stage revival of *A Streetcar Named Desire.* I often wonder what's more tragic—the stars of the studio system who died young or those who grew old and became either shut-ins or carica-tures of themselves. Tallulah Bankhead was only sixty-six when she died, of emphysema, malnutrition, and pneu-monia. Her last words were "Codeine . . . bourbon." When I think of Tallulah Bankhead, I think of how she was known for the cutting quip. She was known as more of a personality than an actress, in a way, befitting the childhood friend of Zelda Fitzgerald. She never really had a defining role on stage or screen. There is that line of hers that I believe that I first read in Louise Brooks's memoirs, "I was raped in the driveway when I was 11. You know darling, it was a terrible experience because we had all that gravel." But I don't mention this to my father, when he calls my daughter Tallulah Bankhead.

HEIRESS

I remember the strange feeling of the temporary office I occupied that semester of a feminist film historian on sabbatical, a professor with the last name of Hearst. It was as if I had decorated it myself, with photographs of some of the same actresses that I had previously stuck to the walls of my apartment when attempting to write a failed book of fictional monologues when I first tried to become a writer, now more than a decade ago. I didn't have much contact with this professor, except the time she left a note asking me not to leave my discarded lunch in her trash can, because of the smell. One day there was a knock on my door, or her door, I should say. It was an elderly classics professor whose office was down the hall, in which he was rumored to live, like a hermit, in that small thatched building on the edge of campus. You do know who she's related to, he says to me, in a way I can only describe as impish, pointing at her nameplate. I humored the old man, making chitchat. But it was too easy, the idea that a film historian could be related to the inspiration for *Citizen Kane*. But I just figured out while looking online that the film professor was married to a grandson of Hearst, so she actually married into the Hearst family. I remember how the black-and-white press photograph of Louise Brooks reading on set taped next to the professor's desk reminded me of the beautiful elegy Brooks wrote about her friend Pepi Lederer, niece to Marion Davies, the actress who was the mistress to William Randolph Hearst. This made me want to go back and reread it, which I finally now have done. The essay is a matryoshka doll of autobiography, as are the other seven essays collected in *Lulu in Hollywood*, published in 1982, a couple of years before her death and a few years after Kenneth Tynan's famous *New Yorker* profile. For the essay, Tynan visits her in her one-bedroom hermitage in Rochester, New York, where she moved in the 1950s after quitting New York, which she quit after quitting Hollywood. Brooks moved to Rochester at the invitation of the curator of the Eastman film archives, in order to watch old movies, including her own, and to write about them and her memories in film. In her essay "Marion Davies' Niece," Brooks writes of her own retirement from Hollywood in 1940, when she first moved back to her father's home in Kansas, and then to New York City, where she realized the best-paying option for an unsuccessful actress at the age of thirty-six was as a call girl. She eventually worked at the counter at Saks for forty dollars a week. "I blacked out my past, refused to see my few remaining friends connected with movies, and began to flirt with fancies related to little bottles filled with yellow sleeping pills." Whether or not Louise Brooks was a call girl, specifically, or whether she was just kept, in a way, by several wealthy men, is unknown, because she never wrote her memoirs, not really, just these essays. In fact, elsewhere, Brooks called her attempts at memoir, in her quippy way, "Incinerator One," and "Incinerator Two." By 1973, Brooks writes, she no longer accepted the Hollywood judgment that condemned her to failure, and began to research writing about her friend Marion Davies's niece, who had been dead by that time for thirty-eight years, having killed herself at twenty-five years old by jumping out of a window at the psychiatric hospital where Hearst and Davies had her committed for her drug addiction. In her essays Louise Brooks is often a satellite revolving around more famous people, like Humphrey Bogart or Charlie Chaplin, much like her friend was always on the margins, cracking jokes at the end of the table at dinners at Hearst Castle, which is where they met. Louise Brooks writes in the essay that she thought when she quit Hollywood she was cured of its disease of fame, but realized that she hadn't been completely cured, because for so long she discounted writing about her friend who committed suicide because she too was viewed as a failure. Her friend Pepi was a party animal, her girlfriend part of Tallulah Bankhead's coterie—that's where Pepi got her coke from. Pepi tried to be a writer for a Hearst magazine as well as an actress and didn't succeed at either, despite her wit and charm. She failed at both. Brooks's essay begins with a meditation on suicide, "No one knows for certain why anyone commits suicide." The day I write this a successful celebrity has just committed suicide. It was the second celebrity this week to have committed suicide, and using the same methods. It's all I can think about the entire day. When did publications begin running parallel articles about how celebrities react on Twitter to tragedies? Why do I always read them? Do these responses make me feel less alone? These two celebrities who committed suicide were extremely accomplished, generous, and loved. How exhausting that labor, to keep that up, all of that success, what everyone must have wanted from them at all times. Success doesn't erase pain or torment. Then what does it do? Is it to have more for us to mourn when they are gone? But what about the failures and the forgotten? Don't they need to be mourned as well?

LOUISE BROOKS IN A
MINT-GREEN HOUSECOAT

Instead of preparing for my Skype interview for a teaching job that was not only low-paying but involved moving overseas to another expensive city we couldn't afford to live in, a job that I was not going to get but also didn't really want, I watched a documentary about Louise Brooks on YouTube. Over the years I have been watching this documentary, a bit at a time. It's all I did today, really, except finally make it to a yoga class and monitor my daughter's diaper rash. I don't know what I did with all of my obsessions before YouTube. When I was trying to write about Louise Brooks over a decade ago, thinking about her almost half century of reclusiveness, I certainly would have wanted to watch this documentary. The filmmakers came to her apartment in 1974, when she was sixty-eight years old, to ask her about her time making two iconic silent films with G. W. Pabst, *Pandora's*

Box and *Diary of a Lost Girl*. These are the films we think of when we think about Louise Brooks, all shiny black bob and creamy slender body, an innocence to her fatality, like Kansas City meets Berlin. The film begins with clips from those films—a movement from her young hands to old hands. She is sitting at her Formica table, a green sofa behind her, and wearing a fairly threadbare mint-green housecoat or robe, her hair now extremely long and almost more green than gray, the bangs grown out, all pulled back in a tight ponytail. She is powdered and has red lipstick on. She is still recognizable—the face now from the face then. The skin, I've started to notice skin—how it becomes thinner, pulls downward. Also, a lifetime of smoking, of being shut inside. It is strange to hear her voice, as most of her films were silent, although I recognized her voice, having watched her in the John Wayne B film *Overland Stage Raiders*, her last role. She has a nice voice—I won't overload it with birdlike adjectives like Kenneth Tynan does in his 1979 *New Yorker* profile, when after watching *Pandora's Box* on cable, the theater critic exiled in Los Angeles and dying of emphysema realizes Brooks is still alive and has been living as a shut-in in Rochester, New York, and sets out on a pilgrimage. Her hands folded on the table, she is stern and certain with her narration. MGM wasn't going to give her a raise with her option—this was in the late '20s; they were going to pay her $750 a week still, to put her in a string of mediocre Hollywood films. Or there was some guy in

Berlin called Pabst who would pay her $1,000 a week to make these other films. So she quit and went to Berlin. And afterwards the head of the studio spread the lie that she left Hollywood because she couldn't make it once talking films were popularized. In his profile Tynan notes that Brooks has not left her apartment since 1960, for more than two decades, except for a few doctor or dentist appointments. When he interviews her, she has been bedridden for some time with osteoarthritis of the hip. He interviews her while she's in bed, as she sifts through old photographs and narrates them, and lights cigarettes. They seem to have fallen in love with each other then, or to be already in love with each other. Apparently they kept up a correspondence afterwards. It's very *Veronika Voss*. She speaks in the monologue of the lonely not used to having real conversation. She says to Tynan, "You're doing a terrible thing to me. I've been killing myself off for twenty years, and you're going to bring me back to life." She spends her life in memories and books, and, he notes, in two rooms, that are clean and modestly furnished. The pathos of the descriptions of the two rooms really gets me, that she is obviously living in genteel poverty, which is made apparent by her shabby mint-green housecoat, which she must have owned for many years. In the large room, Venetian blinds, the green sofa, the table, a TV set, and "flesh-pink walls sparsely hung with paintings redolent of the twenties." In the other room, a single bed, a cupboard filled with press clippings, a set of drawers with the crucifix and Virgin statue on top. And a stool piled with books. The serious authors, Tynan notes—Schopenhauer, Ortega y Gasset, Edmund Wilson, Proust. She insists on getting out of bed to escort him to the door, with her cane, while she mentions how Proust wrote in bed as well. It's true, the asthmatic writer enclosed himself into his cork-filled room, away from noise and dust and cooking smells, and wrote *In Search of Lost Time* over a decade. The fur coat that he didn't take off, regardless of the temperature.

AUTHOR PHOTO, PART THREE

In the recent series of photographs taken on the occasion of her new novel, the famous novelist looks different. It's been several years since the last book came out, so naturally she looks older. She is, after all, no longer the gamine writing about being a young woman. Then, she was in her thirties, writing about being in her twenties. Now, she is forty, writing about her late thirties. There is always a lag in publishing books about one's life. The hope is of course her passionate readers will follow her. Also, she appears to be growing out her distinctive bangs. She was so recognizable before. She is still recognizable, although slightly less recognizable. As she grows out her hair, will she continue to become less and less recognizable? Her book has gotten wonderful reviews. Once again reinventing the form, et cetera.

ELENA FERRANTE

My mother-in-law identifies as a big reader. She loves romances and family dramas. They cannot be, however, too dark. She did not like, for instance, Jonathan Franzen's *The Corrections*. She especially did not like the depiction of the character of the mother in that book. I also dislike the work of Jonathan Franzen, for a variety of reasons, but really I like to think this is where the similarities between our reading habits end. When we visited her in the Detroit suburbs the summer that I was pregnant, I recommended that she read Elena Ferrante. The only Elena Ferrante I had read was *The Days of Abandonment*, which I read while sitting on the porch during a hot summer a few years earlier. I inhaled the book, which I heard happens when you read Elena Ferrante—the books are just that good. I remember there's a moment where the narrator, completely unraveling after her husband leaves her for another woman, trapped alone in her apartment with two small children, writes in her notebook about *Jane Eyre* while sitting on a park bench. I liked that moment the best. Also when the glass shatters in the pasta sauce, because it reminds me of my family. This, I do not say to my mother-in-law, as she would not understand. I tell her to read the Neapolitan Novels, which I haven't read, only because I get annoyed by books that get too much attention and find myself allergic to them. When I go into a bookstore, everyone tells me to read Elena Ferrante, and instead I go read something else. Also people always ask me what I think about Elena Ferrante. Perhaps because I've spoken in interviews about not being on social media anymore, which is also a lie. I am not social on social media anymore, but I still ghost social media. I still look at different accounts and look to see when I'm mentioned. Many of my friends who are writers talk to me often about Elena Ferrante. When we complain about publishing and expected publicity, we say, "Wouldn't it be nice to be Elena Ferrante?" Or: "Elena Ferrante really has it figured out." But what does that mean? Elena Ferrante has figured out how to write commercially successful, critically revered international bestsellers but doesn't have to have people in her life know that she wrote them, or doesn't have to have her picture taken. The publishing industry loves Elena Ferrante—there's no one the publishing industry loves more than Elena Ferrante. They would not love Elena Ferrante's disappearance, or appearance of disappearance, if she did not also write commercial best-sellers that are widely seen as brilliant as well. Let's be real here! It's not that she writes under a pseudonym. She's like Batman, Elena Ferrante. People wouldn't love Batman for his costumed anonymity unless he saved the people of Gotham from villains. People wouldn't love just the costume. The costume is an effect of mystery. But anyway, I had not seen my mother-in-law for some time. I guess you could say we've been estranged, especially since the election. We have only seen them once, since then, when the baby was born and they came to New York, and I recommended they go to Magnolia Bakery, because of *Sex and the City*, because I thought she'd enjoy it, which she did. I recommended Magnolia Bakery like I recommended Elena Ferrante. Both I thought she'd enjoy, and I was right. My mother-in-law had never heard of Elena Ferrante, and so she was immediately suspicious, how I had heard of Elena Ferrante. I was sitting there in her easy chair in her living room, huge in the heat, despite only being six months pregnant, I looked at term, and I was drinking water, and she asked me for reading recommendations. I never know how to respond when people ask me how I hear of writers. And after all, Elena Ferrante is pretty mainstream. I'm sure her books are sold at your Barnes & Noble, I then said to my mother-in-law, which turned out to be true. But how did you know of her, she kept on asking me. Well, I am a writer, I said to her, then, and she still looked perplexed, because my in-laws don't think of me as a writer. I think they think of me as a teacher who can't get a full-time job, which is I think how my father thinks of me as well. This used to bother me, but now this invisibility is its own comfort. I don't have to worry about them reading my writing, so I can write whatever I want. It reminds me of my childhood and adolescence and life, really, so it reminds me why I am a writer in the first place. Although do I write as a form of disappearance, or as a reaction against disappearance? Sometimes I do wonder what level of material success would make my family members or in-laws acknowledge that I'm a real writer, whatever that is. What fellowship or award? But not getting fellowships or awards, it's hard to say. Sometimes I think they have a stake in thinking of me as invisible. This has been helped greatly by having a child and turning forty, because it has allowed me to become even more invisible. Now, they only see and talk about the child, or me in relation to the child. I think that Elena Ferrante became Elena Ferrante so she could write from her life without embarrassing her family or those she loved. Maybe, also, so she didn't have to go through publicity, this ideal of letting the work speak for itself. She didn't have to be an author photo, or to have this author photo scrutinized as she aged. She could truly be faceless. Elena Ferrante could disappear into this name, and this work, so she could have her own name in her life. Names always get in the way, my friend M. said to me. In the way of literature, I think is what she meant. It is not lost on me the irony that publishing insists on making their authors become brands, their photographs taken in style sections and countless interviews, my god all the interviews, and all the essays, and keeping up on Twitter, and being constantly witty and profound, and the events, but they love their Elena Ferrante. Although Elena Ferrante has a column for the *Guardian* now. Not that there's anything wrong with that. Clarice Lispector had a column too, her *cronicas*, which I love. I'm sure my publishers wish I wrote a column somewhere, or did more interviews, or anything anymore, and the truth is I do a little, probably more than some, and get too exhausted or sick of myself speaking, or writing answers, and then stop. It's not that I think I'm so pure; it's that I get too tired. We can only do, I suppose, what we're capable of. I would like not to even have my photograph taken anymore, or use any author photo in the back of any books, or do any events, or anything more than writing books, so maybe if I put that here, maybe that will help make my point. I can't do that, I will say. It's in the book! Maybe I can just say I'm being like Elena Ferrante, and that this lack of publicity is actually a form of publicity, and they'll buy that somehow. Although, again, without writing books that a lot of people want to read, that probably won't work. After reminding my mother-in-law that I was a writer, and that in fact I taught writing, I also told her that Elena Ferrante's works are widely reviewed, in places like the *New York Times*, which she regarded with even more suspicion. Then I told her that bookstores sold her books on the front table, and that she appeared to accept. If you were wondering, my mother-in-law loved the books. She went through all of them, and gave them to her mother and everyone she knew, who also read them and loved them. Everyone, it seems, loves Elena Ferrante. When people ask me about Elena Ferrante, I usually respond that I prefer Elsa Morante, who is Elena Ferrante's favorite writer, and the inspiration for her pseudonym, although in truth I have only read *Aracoeli*, which I did love, but not any more than I loved *The Days of Abandonment*. This is what I really think when I think about Elena Ferrante. I think of this story my father told me a couple years ago, about an aunt who was Neapolitan, and how she finally threw a butcher knife at her cheating abusive husband, and it landed in the door. For some time she left the knife in there, and even after she removed it, she kept the mark that it had created in the door, as a reminder.

THE BARBIZON HOTEL FOR WOMEN

A few years back the sign from the local storage company on the Q train read "You're Not Little Edie, and This Isn't Grey Gardens." Something about this sign, one of those quippy and ubiquitous signs from that company, bothered me. I didn't know exactly what it meant. It felt like a slight at Little Edie, who so longed to move back to New York City, to be by herself, to try to have a chance at "making it." Little Edie who just wanted to go back to the Barbizon. "All I want is a little room . . . Any little rat's nest in New York City . . ." (I'm copying this line from Wayne Koestenbaum's *Hotel Theory*.) Why did Big Edie make her leave the Barbizon? Her mother replied that she thought she'd been in New York long enough . . . She was getting lines on her face. But she didn't want to leave! Edie was at the Barbizon Hotel for Women from 1947 to 1952, right before Sylvia Plath got there for her internship at *Mademoiselle*. The Barbizon becomes the Amazon in *The Bell Jar*. When I had my own magazine internship and nervous breakdown, I stayed at the Webster Apartments in midtown, which was the less famous hotel for women.

I had one friend at the Webster, a girl on a costume fellowship at Juilliard. She got me free tickets to see plays like *The Duchess of Malfi*. I was writing a bad play in my little room. I would stay in every night and write my bad little play and on the weekends walk downtown to Washington Square Park and sit there and read and watch everything. I was so happy and miserable at the same time. I was supposed to room with the costume designer in Astoria once I graduated, but since I didn't move back to New York for fifteen years, it didn't happen.

REPLY ALL

You receive another email from your department head that a tenured faculty member at the college has won a prestigious award. It is one of many awards this writer has won this season. All day your inbox is filled with other faculty, all writers, expressing their congratulations, competing in exclamations. You wonder all day, again, whether a writer is ever truly happy for another writer who wins an award.

SCREEN TESTS

I woke up and watched a video series on the website of a literary magazine that was about writers and their first published books. Each short video portrait was approximately six minutes long, and framed the writer from the torso up. The interviews were intercut with photographs of the writers when they were young and moony, as many of the writers published their first books when they were in their twenties. They were filmed in their living spaces, often against their bookshelves. Often these writers spoke of "making it," or this longing to "make it." (What is "it," exactly? I always want to know.) I was nervous because the camera crew was coming by later in the month to film me, about my first book, which came out on a very small press. I was mostly concerned about where I would sit, and what I would wear, and how I would hold myself to render myself into a talking head.

Later, when the filmmakers came, I found it difficult to sit still and look straight ahead at the person interviewing me, and not at the camera. I wore a black silk dress, and asked if they would shoot me closer up, as I was still nursing and wearing a nursing bra. In a photograph I saw of the film shoot, I look like Liza Minnelli. Not, I should add, Liza Minnelli then, but Liza Minnelli now. Yes, exactly like her. I never knew until I moved here that women writers were expected to be photogenic. I thought this was one of the reasons I became a writer, so that I could be ugly and folded over and inside my head all the time. I didn't realize my jawline had disappeared—it must have happened in the past year. This morning I watch a video for facial yoga. I read the horrible news. Then, in order to calm down, I watch some of Warhol's Screen Tests. The Screen Tests each took three minutes to shoot but then Warhol slowed them to four minutes. The subject was asked to be still for the duration of the reel, but it wasn't possible, to just be their own image. They blink, they breathe, they smoke, they drink a Coke (Lou Reed). The dots that explode after each one at the end of the hundred-foot Bolex reel. Warhol had the idea perhaps he would sell them as living portrait boxes, playing in individual homes. The filmmakers interviewed me for several hours, but they will cut that down into only six minutes, they said. I think I often moved around on my chair, even though I was supposed to stay still, and was probably too animated with my mouth and my gestures. Warhol's favorite Screen Test was apparently Ann Buchanan, the one who cries a single tear. I've watched this one many times, as unlike most of them it's been uploaded online. She looks so contemporary, in her long thick dark hair and thick eyebrows. How can she be so still, despite all the commotion about her, the people filming, watching? She gazes at you and you gaze back. The bare movement of her breathing. The performance of such intensity. What a beautiful face, someone wrote in the comments. Now she should have made it, someone else wrote. Was it a trick she could perform, that single tear falling?

EDIE FILM

Edie Sedgwick met Andy Warhol at a birthday party for Tennessee Williams. She grew up on a California ranch. Her father was an artist who wanted his children to call him Fuzzy. When Warhol met Edie, her hair was in a beehive and her leg was in a cast. She had already been in psych wards on the East Coast. She studied art at Cambridge and spent a year making a sculpture of a horse. She was twenty-one years old. She had just received her trust fund. The year earlier two of her brothers had committed suicide. They were suicidal heirs, like the Wittgensteins, but from Massachusetts. Soon she made her hair a helmet like Warhol's, with silver spray. When he invited her to Paris, she wore a white mink and packed a suitcase with another white mink. Edie Sedgwick made ten movies with Andy Warhol in 1965, ending with 1966's *Lupe*, apparently inspired by Kenneth Anger's account of the suicide of Lupe Vélez. Warhol wanted to make a movie where Edie commits suicide at the end. Apparently he also wondered out loud whether Edie would in fact commit suicide someday, and if so, if she would let Warhol film it. After breaking up with Andy, Edie lived at the Chelsea Hotel with Bob Dylan, then was in and out of institutions for the rest of the 1960s, and finally overdosed on barbiturates. Lupe Vélez also overdosed, as did Marilyn Monroe. Was Warhol drawn to Edie because she was his Marilyn, or was Warhol his own Marilyn? I have read reviews of the Edie films and read about them in Douglas Crimp's book and watched minute-long clips, which are these out-of-focus corners of nothingness. It's almost impossible to find a Warhol film online—you have to catch a screening somewhere. In *Lupe*, like the other Edie films, Warhol films Edie smoking and hanging around her apartment, not as Lupe but as Edie Sedgwick. Warhol's Edie films were about Edie Sedgwick. They were portraits, like his paintings, but with time added. There's nothing Edie does to impersonate someone else. She only impersonates Edie Sedgwick.

NICO IN THE KITCHEN
CUTTING HER BANGS

Could I write this text rendered in split screen, with the sound only on one side, like in Warhol's *Chelsea Girls*? The beginning of the film, on the right, Nico is in the kitchen cutting her bangs. So often there's haircutting in Warhol movies. Factory photographer Billy Name was the son of a Poughkeepsie barber. He starred in *Haircut 1, 2,* and *3*. He also cuts Edie Sedgwick's hair in *Lupe*. It was Ray Johnson who brought Andy Warhol to one of Billy Name's haircut parties—that's how they met. The walls were covered in silver foil. Can you, Warhol asked, do that for my loft?

MEG RYAN VEHICLE

When I was in college in the late '90s, I was obsessed with the movie *Addicted to Love* starring Meg Ryan. It is a lesser-known 1997 Meg Ryan vehicle, with some resemblance in story structure to *French Kiss*, which came out two years earlier, although the gender roles are somewhat reversed. Amazing to realize that *Addicted to Love* came out just a year before *You've Got Mail*. Both of these Meg Ryan movies helped form my conception of New York, but Meg Ryan is Upper West Side in *You've Got Mail*, and more bourgeois and seemingly older. She's only in her mid-thirties in both of these films. The style however is totally different. In *You've Got Mail*, she is the classic turtleneck-and-sweater-set Meg Ryan. I remember watching *You've Got Mail* and not knowing how anyone could have her life together enough to wear such a series of prim stone-colored knits and linens. In *Addicted to*

Love, which is named after the Robert Palmer song, Meg Ryan is still Meg Ryan, and still has the classic shaggy bob, but she is a more downtown Meg Ryan. I was obsessed with Meg Ryan's style in this movie. Her bleached bob with skunk roots that Sally Hershberger would hack pieces out of in a just-so way, where she looks like an extremely expensive and glamorous wreck. I read a partial chapter online on Meg Ryan's hair in *Addicted to Love* in a book on the films of Meg Ryan. Meg Ryan needed Hershberger on set, because not anyone could hack into that Meg Ryan hair. It actually took a lot of work, for the Meg Ryan bob to be deconstructed in such a specific way. I think that *Addicted to Love* was Meg Ryan's first role where she tried to not be so Meg Ryan. Watching it, now, I feel even then she wanted to break out somehow of the Meg Ryan character. I probably watch the movie once a year. It's my favorite bad film. Matthew Broderick plays a small-town astronomer with a daily noon ritual of watching his schoolteacher fiancée, played by a sundressed Kelly Preston, from his telescope, which is supposed to be romantic. When she leaves him and moves to Manhattan, he cashes out his life savings to, basically, stalk her, squatting in an abandoned building across the way from the apartment of her new lover, a sexy French chef. Broderick's character creates a camera obscura so that he can monitor and watch all of their goings-on as projected on a screen like a real-time film. Now, watching the movie, I recognize the Wooster Street address in Soho where the French chef and the Kelly Preston character live as the beautiful cast-iron building that in real life houses the Drawing Center. Meg Ryan plays the vaguely Diane Arbus–like photographer (she alludes to taking photographs of freakish types, but also makes collages on a wall that badly approximate Barbara Kruger exclamations). She rides around on a motorcycle at the beginning of the film, like a Fury seeking vengeance on the French chef who married her just for the green card. Eventually, she crashes Matthew Broderick's pad, and collaborates with him on ruining the chef's life. And in the process, of course, they fall in love. At the beginning of the film Meg Ryan tries to not be Meg Ryan; she skulks around, all sullen rage, her bleached hair and raccoon smoky eyes. When I watched this film in college, I thought all of the outfits she wore were the epitome of cool. Recently, when watching it on my laptop, I took pictures of all of her looks on my phone. The motorcycle goggles and maroon leather jacket with shearling collar, that blue-green feather boa (I got one in college to look just like it), the red tank dress underneath. The quilted patterned robe with the belt. The burgundy tank with yellow stripes and a black miniskirt. The red velvet smoking blazer paired with leopard print. That red velvet blazer now with a leather bandanna, as she takes photographs in Washington Square Park. (Meg Ryan isn't really the one taking the photographs, the camera is actually gazing at her, we are looking at her.) I think a more sophisticated version of this film could have been a commentary on watching, and the gaze, and moviemaking itself, but it doesn't get there. All of these shots I take on my phone remind me of Edie Sedgwick's Screen Test, how there's magnetism to her even though she's just looking. The vibrato to her breathing. When Meg Ryan was preparing for *Addicted to Love*, she was thinking about Edie Sedgwick as well, studying a book about her to think at least about the style elements, but the film is not boring in an interesting way like an Andy Warhol movie, or dark like Edie Sedgwick's story. It is ultimately conventional. The movie begins in one way, but by the end becomes a Meg Ryan vehicle, if a less successful Meg Ryan vehicle because she tamps down her Meg Ryan exuberance for most of the film. People want to see Meg Ryan cranky, but cranky in a quirky way. Toward the end, she loosens up and becomes cuddly again, in that Meg Ryan way. She still has that Meg Ryan smile. She's not so tough after all, despite her smoky eyes and leather jacket. It's like Ally Sheedy in *The Breakfast Club*—the scowl comes with the makeup, but there's softness underneath. There's Meg Ryan laughing. There's Meg Ryan looking at Matthew Broderick with that Meg Ryan look. She's lit so well. Meg Ryan and that quirk of her nose, the range of its expressiveness. Meg Ryan hurt. Meg Ryan in love. Meg Ryan pining. Meg Ryan hurt again. Meg Ryan annoyed. Meg Ryan sad. Meg Ryan thoughtful. Meg Ryan kissing Matthew Broderick with an open mouth. No one kisses like '90s-era Meg Ryan, so totally open and going for it, like she's going to eat his face. The day I started rewatching this film Meg Ryan was in the news again. A producer accused Harvey Weinstein of jacking off in front of her in a theater while they were screening a nude Meg Ryan scene from *In the Cut*. Her string of failures after these hits in the '90s. Meg Ryan trying to step out of being Meg Ryan. *Addicted to Love* was also a failure. People want Meg Ryan's face to do Meg Ryan things. And now, Meg Ryan has done something to her face. What has Meg Ryan done to her face? You can watch many slideshows online, about Meg Ryan's changing face. Meg Ryan is not Meg Ryan anymore. Meg Ryan is still alive, but she is not frozen in time. Meg Ryan is supposed to stay Meg Ryan, that Meg Ryan, no, that Meg Ryan.

ANDY WARHOL SELF-PORTRAIT

One of my daughter's favorite books is an Andy Warhol children's book called *Andyland: The Art and Wisdom of Andy Warhol*. It was one of her favorite books as a little baby and now that she's a year older she still loves it. You turn the pages for one of Andy Warhol's silk screen paintings and a word—"Flowers," "Boat," "Heart," "Beauty," "People," "Banana," "Art"—and you can flip up the word to reveal one of Warhol's koan-like musings. (Banana: "You need to let the little things that would ordinarily bore you suddenly thrill you.") The last opening is of the word "You" across from a version of one of Andy Warhol's 1986 self-portraits but rendered as a mirrored silhouette against a black background. My daughter's favorite part of the book is this page, as she can look at her reflection. I have several photos on my phone of her baby face looking through the Andy Warhol self-portrait. Although my daughter doesn't really understand yet what "you" means or what "I" means or what "me" means. This week we're trying to teach her her own name. It's still wavy, concepts of boundaries and identity for her. Every time lately we get to that last page—which is at least once a day—and there's that moment of my daughter merging with the blank reflection of Andy Warhol, I think about how strange it is, to have in a children's book a mirrored silhouette of one of Andy Warhol's 1986 self-portraits that were playing with the plasticity of his fright wig. How haunting and empty those self-portraits are, like a death mask. How Andy Warhol was never the same after Valerie Solanas shot him. Billy Name has said afterwards he was like "Cardboard Andy." My daughter also loves listening to David Bowie's song "Andy Warhol," which makes me think of how years later David Bowie played Warhol all wig and emptiness in Julian Schnabel's biopic of *Basquiat*. How uncanny that performance is. Sometimes when I think about Andy Warhol, I'm really thinking about David Bowie playing Andy Warhol. Andy Warhol by the time period of this late self-portrait was also playing Andy Warhol. In an interview with Billy Name, now seventy-two, at *The New Yorker*, in answer to his favorite memory from his time with Warhol, he answers that it was when Andy was shot. It is such a strange answer. It's almost like he needs to talk about it.

He came out of the darkroom and Andy was shot and everyone was in shock. Andy was in a pool of blood. He held him and started crying, and Andy said, "Oh, Billy, don't make me laugh, it hurts too much." In answer to his worst memory from that time, Billy Name says it's still when Andy was shot. It's the same memory, he says.

TWO

As I am just finishing an application for a grant I will not get, I noticed that one of last year's recipients was a theater director from Chicago. He won the grant for his twenty-two-hour cycle of extant ancient Greek drama. I felt a prick of panic or shame, when I read this, as I had interviewed this director fifteen years ago for the publication I worked for at the time, but never filed the story, as my mother was dying, and I moved home to take care of her. I remember how young and sure of himself he was, and I remember feeling I would never be an artist like that, that it seemed impossible to me. I always felt badly about that—that he arranged to meet me in person, as that's what we did then, and we talked for an hour or two, which I recorded, and then never transcribed. What a waste of time that was for him, I imagine. In that same period I also interviewed a well-known male memoirist who was in town for a festival. We met at the lobby of his hotel. I remember he asked me if I wanted to go upstairs to his room to finish the interview. I declined. I also didn't file that interview, but don't feel bad about that. Since I moved here, I saw him at one of the three parties I have attended in the past five years, and he hit on me again, but didn't connect that I was also that young journalist in the lobby of a Michigan Avenue hotel. Why should he? Anyway, perhaps I wasn't that person—maybe I just shared the same name as that person. Although he was evidently the same.

DIANE ARBUS VISITS MARILYN MINTER IN GAINESVILLE, FLORIDA

Marilyn Minter was a photography student at the University of Florida, in Gainesville, in 1969. She had just shown her fellow students the proof sheets from a series of black-and-white photographs of her mother, a glamorous drug addict and recluse, taken when visiting her one weekend at the Coral Ridge Towers, an apartment complex near Fort Lauderdale. The photographs look like stills out of a late Joan Crawford or Bette Davis movie. A glamorous woman in a wig wearing a negligee stares at a gilded mirror. She is in bed, surrounded by bottles of pills, rather languidly smoking. Her daughter took twelve shots, one roll of 2¼-inch film. Her fellow students were horrified that this was her mother. Diane Arbus was a visiting artist at the time, and praised the proof sheets when she saw them. Minter remembers Arbus wearing a silver minidress, silver sandals, short hair, and no bra. No one dressed like that in Florida. She didn't know then that Arbus was a famous artist, or what about these photographs would have drawn her in. Looking at them now, it makes sense. There's something both cruel and tender about the gaze. A way of encountering her mother in her claustrophobic element. Despite the lone encouragement of an alien visitor, Marilyn Minter didn't print the photographs for years, so depressed by her peers' critiques. What was Sontag's issue with Arbus in her book on photography, her critique that her photographs lacked empathy? After all, who can be crueler than critics? I saw these Coral Ridge Towers photographs at the Marilyn Minter retrospective at the Brooklyn Museum a couple years ago. They were the first photographs you saw, on the wall, when you walked in. I recognized something in how haunted and isolated her mother looked in those pictures, and yet defiant among her cosmetics and pills. I could have stared forever. I was heavily pregnant, almost two weeks overdue. My midwife had told me to go do something fun, to take my mind off of things. While I was there I ran into a famous editor, who had worked with Kathy Acker and David Wojnarowicz and Karen Finley, and who had edited an essay I wrote in an anthology. She was with a friend of hers who had written the definitive book on ACT UP. We embraced, but she eyed me nervously.

She seemed worried I was going to go into labor right then, that my water would break all over the museum floor. We'll all be stuck here all night, she said. That's not how it works, I wanted to say to her, but didn't. It's not like in the movies.

VALERIE SOLANAS IN A SILVER LAMÉ DRESS

There's a detail in the Valerie Solanas biography that I find so compelling—that after the long decade in and out of psych wards and on and off of the streets after she shot Warhol, she moved to San Francisco in the '80s, the final three years of her life, and was spotted in the Tenderloin district in a silver lamé dress. Also that the biographer gleaned this detail from an essay entitled "Valerie Solanas in a Silver Lamé Dress" that the New Narrative writer Bruce Boone wrote for a Valerie Solanas–themed zine. In the mid-'90s Bruce Boone went to the single-occupancy welfare hotel in San Francisco and interviewed two middle-aged sex workers in the lobby who remembered Valerie, who by that time wasn't going by "Valerie Solanas" anymore, but by some other name. "The hotel lobby was dispiriting," Bruce Boone writes. "I mean, here was this woman who had this New York life—the go-go years, Warhol and that crowd, whatever—and in her minor maybe but real way famous—in this hellhole of a welfare pit of a hotel. There was the heartbreak of having to know how a great spirit ended, totally unknown too, and just a hooker (just!) after being Valerie." This is quoted in the biography. I couldn't get a hold of the essay or the zine—I wrote to the person who published the zine, actually a series of Solanas-themed zines, who was a librarian in Nebraska, and he wrote back but didn't have any copies left, and I also wrote to Bruce Boone, but never heard back. I'm sure he's busy. The women told Bruce Boone that they remember Valerie as slim and elegant, in that great silver lamé dress she loved. But there were other reports of her covered in scabs, addicted to meth. Someone remembers seeing her in her room in those last days, typing away at her desk with her manual typewriter, pages everywhere, writing furiously into the night. The Solanas biography had just come out when I moved to the city, and I went to a conversation about it at Bluestockings with my friend Clutch. I think this might have been the first time I ever hung out with them. We met up with Jackie Wang. I remember, I was wearing this long white shirt over black skinny jeans, and a leather jacket, and a vintage men's little black Comme des Garçons hat, and heavy eye makeup, and a heavy white bronze necklace, like a choker, that I had bought at a boutique, and returned later, because it was turning my neck green. I guess that was my costume when I moved here. I wanted to look like a pretty boy who was also a pickpocket and an art bitch. Anyway, we sat cross-legged in back, and I raised my hand during the Q&A and asked whether the biographer thought that Valerie was really working on something. And what happened to this manuscript? I've always romanticized the possibilities of it, despite many reports of Valerie Solanas's increasing paranoia, like Robert Walser writing microscripts with a pencil while at Waldau. A novel in Swedish by Sara Stridsberg speculates about Valerie's last days, but it hasn't been translated into English. The biographer didn't seem optimistic that Valerie Solanas was seriously writing or that what she was writing was serious. Above all she wanted to be taken seriously as a writer. There were always sightings of Valerie in the '60s and '70s in New York—Valerie sleeping on park benches, hanging around St. Marks, spending days drifting, in and out of cheap hotels, the Chelsea Hotel and the Hotel Earle, where she stayed in the wing for drag queens and lesbians, along with Candy Darling. In her story on Valerie in *Airless Spaces*, Shulamith Firestone writes about visiting her in her new apartment, how nice it was, the Doric columns outside of the building. Valerie talked about how the Mob had put a transmitter in her uterus to follow her. Shulie, herself in and out of psych wards, wondered if maybe Valerie was correct in her delusions that she was being followed. She observes that Valerie was still dressed in a bohemian costume: her little white socks, her collar up, "always a poor girl chic." There are differing reports of what Valerie Solanas was wearing on June 3, 1968, when she shot Andy Warhol. Was her hair combed? Did she wear mascara, lipstick? A dress? A yellow or black turtleneck? A blue one? A yellow sweatshirt? A yellow blouse or yellow trousers? Tennis shoes or torn sneakers without socks? A trench coat? In her bag a gun, an address book, a menstrual pad. After the shooting, Andy Warhol described the thick web of scars on his torso as covering him like a Dior dress.

WITTGENSTEIN'S MISTRESS

It doesn't seem believable Kate could get laid, said my graduate student. We had been reading David Markson's *Wittgenstein's Mistress*. Is it because, I asked, she is the last person on earth, or because you think she's old, or because you think she's crazy? He seemed to think all of it. I'm sure she did just fine, I said to him, rather defensively. Whenever I think about *Wittgenstein's Mistress*, I think about my roommate way back when, who I've written about before, who was a decade older than me and in love with a literary scholar a decade older than she who had written an important (apparently) scholarly essay on that book. How when he broke up with her, so cruelly, she locked herself in her room and lived in her bed like a shipwreck on an island. I was a waitress then. Years later I sat across from him in Bergen, Norway, as I had accompanied my spouse to a literary conference. He had no idea of the connection, I'm sure. He looked like a well-slicked mole man. I watched him slurp his soup and speak about the contemporary American novel and I hated him in sympathy for my former friend. This sort of heavily referential writing is difficult for readers, I've been told. Bricolage, Kate said.

HENRY FOOL

Strange that her favorite movie was Hal Hartley's *Henry Fool*. I've watched this 1997 parable of literary success and failure, a sort of stilted noir, many times since then. When I watch it, I think of her watching it. James Urbaniak plays Simon, the selectively mute garbage man, who encounters Thomas Jay Ryan's criminal janitor Henry Fool, who moves into the garden apartment of the building in Queens where Simon lives with his suicidal mother and his sister, a skinny, jangly Parker Posey. Henry brings in his suitcases his "Confessions," his life's work kept in composition notebooks. "It's a philosophy. A poetics. A politics if you will. A literature of protest. A novel of ideas. A pornographic magazine of truly comic-book proportions. It is in the end whatever the hell I want it to be and when I'm through it's going to blow a hole into the world's idea of itself," Henry explains to

Simon while unloading his notebooks. Simon takes an empty black-and-white composition notebook and, staying up all night in the kitchen, writes an epic poem that goes on to win the Nobel Prize. My former roommate had the same Formica table, I am remembering. Simon reads his mentor's confessions and realizes they're not any good. "He's kind of an exile, marginalized on account of his ideas," he says to his sister, in Henry's defense, earlier. I had the same IBM ThinkPad as Simon that weighed a ton. I wrote capsule-sized theater reviews but wanted to be an avant-garde playwright back then, like Sarah Kane. Both James Urbaniak and Thomas Jay Ryan were actors with Richard Foreman's troupe before they were in *Henry Fool*. It's strange that Parker Posey was in *You've Got Mail* just the year afterward. Such different tonalities. I wonder whether my friend, who I met while working at the coffee shop, who had never finished college and worked a string of dead-end jobs, had wanted to be a writer. Is that why this was her favorite movie? And then I guess I became the writer. Am I the Simon-level fraud or the Henry Fool exile who is also a fraud? Or neither? Or both? Maybe in another dimension she became the writer. I looked for her online again and saw that she started and abandoned a Goodreads account a few years ago. There are ten books on it. Mostly books about Tibetan Buddhism, which is not surprising. But also she wanted to read a Ray Bradbury noir, which kind of is.

GLEANING

I've been meditating, in a rather wandering way, on the history of art as a continuous act of copying. When I had previously watched Agnès Varda's cinematic essay *The Gleaners and I*, I always moved quickly past her opening play with Jean-François Millet's painting *The Gleaners*. I had only been marginally interested in Millet because of van Gogh's yellow-hued copies of his work, the twenty-one canvases of homage painted while at the Saint-Paul asylum; he had no models in the winter, so he painted, after Millet, these studies of piety and light. Varda focuses on the painting for the first minute of her film: she narrates the opening, her cat stares at the camera and nuzzles her old encyclopedia, open to the letter *G*, illustrated with a black-and-white copy of *The Gleaners*—the reproduced, miniature image the filmmaker grew up seeing. "A gleaner is one who gleans," she tells us. That in the past it was only women who gleaned (as in the Millet, whose original title is in the feminine, *Des glaneuses*), although the contemporary gleaners and collectors she focuses on in this film—this meditation on collecting and filmmaking—are both men and women. Pausing the Varda film streaming on my computer, I watch a cheesy online video of the painting in its gold frame, with the closed-captioning on. Piano Muzak. Two subdued radio voices. Millet's painting was a scandal during the 1857 Salon. After the 1848 revolution, Parisians were fearful of the poverty of the countryside, of the peasants being radicalized. Man: "It's an oddly soft painting." Woman: "The colors are muted." Man: "And the brush is not tight, right? There are no hard lines." Woman: "That's true." I never would have looked at this painting more if Varda hadn't made me see it. I return to Varda's shot of the original hanging in the Musée d'Orsay: a man's head in front of the painting, enclosed by the gilded frame. The camera stands still, time elapses: people are looking, pausing; a group, then only an individual; some take pictures in front with cameras (not yet iPhones), quickly snapping away yet refusing to look. We go from a close-up of the painting's three women to the present-day French countryside, a woman in an apron in a harvested field being interviewed by Varda: she mimes how she and her family used to glean ears of wheat, gathering them up in her apron, before the efficiency of modern machines that leave almost nothing behind. Varda notes that the solitary reality of gleaners is in contrast to the collectivity often depicted in paintings of them. She finds one exception, Jules Breton's *Woman Gleaning*, a woman posing with wheat across her shoulder. The filmmaker poses beside the painting with her own wheat, which she then playfully drops and replaces with her handheld camera. The metaphor of the film's original title, *Les glaneurs et la glaneuse*. "There's another woman gleaning in this film, *c'est moi*."

SCREAM TESTS

Whenever I say "Screen Tests," my one-and-a-half-year-old daughter thinks I'm saying "scream," not "screen," and proceeds to enact her best impression of Janet Leigh being stabbed to death in *Psycho*. After shooting the film, Janet Leigh only took baths, never showers.

ESSAYS
(2012–2014)

SLEEPLESS NIGHTS

I have not been writing like I am supposed to, but I have been watching a lot of things on YouTube, which I tell myself counts as writing. I wander around on the Internet, mostly fixated on underground drag performers from the '80s and '90s who performed at places like the Pyramid Club. I like thinking of the small screen on my laptop like a kinetic Joseph Cornell shadow box that manages to contain the exquisite and absurd fury of Ethyl Eichelberger, pouring catharsis into her accordion as Clytemnestra: that red shock wig, the psychotic raccoon eyes, the almost ethereal lavender ball gown. There are only fragments of Ethyl performing online—glitches, moments—shot from the audience. This makes what you can view all the more poignant. The performances have not been archived, have been allowed to disappear—performance itself is so much about disappearance, about the urgency and ephemerality of the present tense, the scratchy video recording—if it exists—documenting a haunting.

*

As Ethyl too is gone. As so many of these performers are gone, so now much of that moment is gone. And it's strange even having videos to watch now. When I first learned of that period of radical art making and living, of refusing to conform, of wild theatrical happenings— first read Cookie Mueller's book and learned about David Wojnarowicz and Ethyl and Karen Finley in Cynthia Carr's collected *Village Voice* columns—all I had were black-and-white pictures, Peter Hujar's beautiful series of his friend Ethyl, leggy sexy Ethyl laughing as Minnie the Maid, Ethyl applying makeup, Ethyl as Nefertiti, Ethyl in a Fashion Pose, Ethyl without drag looking straight at the camera. I had to imagine the performances, the urgency issuing from an open mouth.

*

I had to imagine Anohni stomping around the Lower East Side in combat boots and a black slip, "FUCK YOU" scrawled on her forehead. There's one photograph online of the gothy costumes from when the Blacklips Performance Cult put on *Our Lady of the Flowers*, which seems like everything I wanted experimental theater to be, art to be: psychotic, feral, everything I dreamed about when I was younger, and still dream about. I was doing an interview for a zine the other day, and we started rhapsodizing about *Our Lady of the Flowers*, how Genet wrote the book on scraps of paper that kept getting taken from him. He kept on, madly scrawling inscriptions against this disappearance. The torn-out pictures of his criminals he put on the wall—a model for obsession, everything I write to.

*

The person who cuts my hair now is a former drag queen who, the other day, told me he was reading *Our Lady of the Flowers*. I don't love how he cuts my hair, but I have to keep going to him. He has a deep love and understanding of old Hollywood and glamour. And he's reading Genet. How could I stop going to him?

*

There is an eight-minute film on YouTube that I keep on watching. The film called *Last Address*, directed by Ira Sachs, is mostly silent except for birds chirping, atmospheric street sounds. Steady shot of a New York City building for a few moments, then we are told the name of the downtown artist who died of AIDS who had that as their last address, and what the address was, and then the camera lingers longer on the building. Cookie Mueller, Ethyl Eichelberger, Keith Haring. My eyes fill up at Arthur Russell's address. The other day I was telling John that to me the most beautiful writing would feel like Russell's *World of Echo*, that I want to write how *World of Echo* makes me feel: kind of full and shattered at the same time. The intimacy of this recording. That captures the sound of a body in a room (his voice, his cello) and distorts it with echo, with melancholy.

*

When I moved here, I wandered over to Shulamith Firestone's last address, and looked up to the fifth floor, and stood there for what felt like forever.

*

I told myself that I was going to write about rage today, but instead, I'm writing about elegy. Can one write both with rage and elegy?

*

What I want to write are portraits of my obsessions. But they exist as portraits in my head. Can I focus on each portrait and ask you to meditate upon each one, on the heartache of their disappearance? The glittering elegy to Billie Holiday that Elizabeth Hardwick writes in *Sleepless Nights*, a section that I both love and am deeply ambivalent about. How she appropriates this tortured genius as a deity, not a person. In the same section she documents her friendship with the jazz-obsessed now-dead gay boy, also from Kentucky, a friendship as violent as a love affair—their haunting the jazz clubs. Her remembrances of living at the Hotel Schuyler for transients, drifters, performers. Hardwick, when crafting the novel, studied not only Renata Adler's *Speedboat* but also Rilke's *Notebooks of Malte Laurids Brigge*, and a similar decreation occurs in the work—going away from the self, preferring to tell other stories, of the washerwomen of her youth, of the denizens of the hotel, as opposed to telling her own. An elegy to youth, to a time in New York.

*

For some reason, now I'm thinking about this beautiful cabaret singer I knew during my *Time* magazine internship, my *Bell Jar* days, the prodrome. She had OCD, diagnosed by psychiatrist parents. She gave me advice for battling disturbing thoughts—if you keep on thinking a man is going to come out around the corner and rape and murder you, make it a hundred men. Make it more and more, until it becomes absurd. She also taught me how to take the subway, and the perfect shade of drugstore red. I think she wanted our red lips pressed up against each other's, but it never happened. I really loved being around her. I tried to look her up several years ago, but I couldn't remember her last name.

*

I thought about the play I was trying to write then, when I was exiting the subway at Times Square the other day. I don't know why that memory was triggered, if it's because I used to wander around Times Square at night during that first stint in New York. But I felt very humane and affectionate to this former self. I thought to myself: Perhaps it's our failures, not our successes, that make us artists.

*

I look at Ethyl Eichelberger's Wiki page, and see that Ethyl grew up in a shit town in Illinois, like I grew up in a shit town in Illinois. And that Ethyl went to Knox College (I can even see in my head: the brochure for Knox College) before getting a scholarship to study performing arts in New York. I think one of the reasons I'm so drawn to these queer and radical artists is that so many came from rather dreary and even abusive backgrounds (the kinship between Peter Hujar and David Wojnarowicz), from split-level shit homes in some suburb, from lower-middle-class or working-class backgrounds where nothing was expected of them, who didn't eat at restaurants growing up. Since I moved to New York, I have felt like an outsider among most of the writers I've met here, even the ones I teach. They grew up in families that expected them to do things; they grew up with art and assurances of their creativity. I needed to find artists who were escaping their backgrounds, like I felt I've always been escaping mine—those who have had to work shit jobs, who have hustled too. Who created art against—not art for.

*

For a while I wanted to be a mime. My first trip to Europe was at twenty-one, the metallic living statues at Sacré-Coeur. The year everything began to crack. I would look at photographs I took of those street performers, and thinking about them would make me feel like something broke open. There was something so beautiful about them, how they would be still and mocking for tourists. I wondered what it would be like to make a life out of a theatrical silence. Puppets and mimes and avant-garde theater. Those were my passion. After another pitch to the arts editor at the paper about a local mime troupe, he said to me, amused, Why are you so enthralled by loathed and vanishing art forms?

Of course, now I attempt to write literature.

*

The girl I dragged with me to Paris, on our newly opened credit cards. The second time I had ever flown on a plane. Cheery, Irish-Catholic, South Side. A compulsive liar. Father was a con artist and gambler. She followed me everywhere for a while; we lived together in the city; we waited tables together at the chain pizza restaurant, the one where you had to mention two appetizers by name upon greeting. I still remember the computer codes. Spinach Artichoke Dip: 212. Sesame Ginger Chicken Dumplings: 202.

She's dead now. Suicide at twenty-five. She signed her suicide note with a smiley face. That's the kind of girl she was. She wanted to make sure everyone else was okay. For a while she had it figured out whatever disorder they decided—the meds, the therapy. I was the one who was worried over when we knew each other, which hadn't been for a while. At her wake all these whispers about how she got into the bad drugs. How she slept on the streets. How she supported her addiction. In the coffin, her family dressed her in a long flowery dress, like Laura Ashley. There were all of those horrible posters of photographs of her smiling. But she was always smiling, didn't they realize that, she was always smiling. Her ex-boyfriend, who used to be a jungle DJ, asked after my welfare. I'm a writer now, I told him. I'm fine. I'm still not sure, thinking back, whether I was lying.

*

She was a psychology major. Aren't they always? I was so depressed the whole time in Paris, feeling so vulgar and American—I wanted to wander around the streets and the museums, smoking and feeling alternatively hostile and melancholy. She wanted to drink and go to clubs. But we were still friends, weren't we, we lived together afterwards. And what did we have in common? I don't know.

She was the one who would swoop down and save all of us, the one who seemed to have everything together. The mom type. She would drive us everywhere. When I sublet that place, with all of the heavy furniture, and I would leave the bowls of dried ramen piled up for weeks, and I would sit in that chair and drink whisky and smoke cigarettes, and still refuse to sleep, she was the only one who checked in on me, who took care of me. She would do my laundry with such cheerful briskness.

*

I feel so sure I'm over this—over her death. We both came from the lower-middle-class Chicago suburbs; we were both, despite everything, good Midwestern girls. It took me so long to cure myself of that.

For there is almost no logic, that I survived and she did not. But, also, it seems so strange that I was ever that person. But there must be some connection. But also, sometimes, strange, that I am apparently the person I am now.

*

I could say: she became darker. But I don't know if that's true. She kept doing drugs, and then I stopped. Maybe it's that she buried the darkness underneath so much artificial light. Even those who loved her, they never felt they knew her; there was always something about her, where you didn't even know if she told the truth to herself.

*

The skinny artist boy whose apartment I sublet in my senior year, upon returning from New York, above the buffalo chicken place. He collected boxes of tinfoil; they were in every drawer of the kitchen, the living room. I think he did something with the tinfoil, but I didn't ask what. I kept them there the entire year—I didn't know what you put in drawers, why not tinfoil? When I came over to sign the sublease, we made out on the leather sofa—how did he have such expensive things? They must have been from his parents. I liked his jumpy energy. I think we argued with each other and wrestled around, and no one got off, because for me, it was never about getting off, but about the electricity of the strange collision. I don't think we were even attracted to each other. It was just something to do. The temporary clanging together of two fucked-up people. Most of my intense interactions in the past were like the camaraderie between mental patients. The camaraderie between people who drifted in and out, because that's what people like us did.

*

Also on that leather couch, the closeted avant-garde composer. It was the '90s: all the work was about failure, about glitchy tape recordings. He would leave me long, whining messages on my voicemail, about everything he did and ate that day. He never asked about me, even though I was falling apart. I was the girl who listened— although I didn't really listen, I just didn't say anything back. I was working three jobs—at the Cajun place, at the more run-down pizza joint, at the arts camp during the day. He took me to see post-rock shows in the city, right near where I would later live, was dismayed I was unimpressed. I think I once let him climb on top of me, rather sloppily and disappointingly. I think we kept our clothes on. It didn't matter to me. I was in love with someone else; I think he was too.

*

The essay I've been promising a journal I'd write is on David Wojnarowicz's photographic series of Rimbaud in New York, where he had friends pose in front of the piers, other haunts, wearing a Rimbaud mask. I have been reading biographies for this essay I can't write: C. Carr's new biography, many Rimbaud biographies. Do you have any idea how many biographies of Rimbaud there are, how many biographies of Rimbaud in Africa? Chris Kraus had told me to read this biography about Rimbaud in Africa for the book I wrote for her, and I never did, but I read a couple afterwards, and I think I read the wrong ones.

*

Facts I seize from the biography: That David Wojnarowicz worked at a Pottery Barn. That he died at thirty-seven like Rimbaud. That they were born a century apart. Why Rimbaud? Why always Rimbaud? I don't know. But maybe this: that Rimbaud was allowed to escape his lower-middle-class drudgery, his fate as the perfect schoolboy, by deciding he was a seer, a poet. By building a religion for art made out of suffering, out of experience. That one could become—and then one could disappear. That all of that pain and suffering—that one's childhood—can be for something.

*

Wojnarowicz said to a reporter that he decided to make his Rimbaud in New York series because "I felt, at that time, that I wanted it to be the last thing I did before I ended up back on the streets or died or disappeared." The photographs too feel like grainy ghosts. Mocking apparitions. As if Rimbaud were sighted at a diner. As if David Wojnarowicz were still somehow alive.

*

To go out with anger—to trace one's own disintegration, or disappearance, as he does in *Close to the Knives*, his gorgeous elegy to his dead friend Peter Hujar that also mourns his own dying and fragile body. That has decided not on peace, but on rage. His "blood-filled egg" he carried around with him, an inscribed body. His "memoir of disintegration."

*

That haunting Peter Hujar photograph of Candy Darling on her deathbed. She has the beauty of a consumptive—tranquil and yet feverish. Her makeup perfectly on. The David Wojnarowicz photograph of a shrunken Peter Hujar on his deathbed, Hujar like a medieval saint. In her life Candy Darling transformed herself into a blonde Hollywood starlet—the performance perfect, intact. My favorite part of her documentary, which I recently watched, is the scene in which Candy mimes a Janet Leigh monologue, knowing all of the words.

*

Peter Hujar, who felt an artist should be able to make up their own biography.

*

Je est une autre. "I am another." Rimbaud's famous declaration. When one writes, one is already somebody else. The fiction of the self. Like Elizabeth Hardwick tweaking how many siblings she has in *Sleepless Nights*. Don't pretend to know. But also, the idea that to write, to make art, can allow for transformation.

*

In a recent interview, I was asked to name a book I thought should be remembered, and I chose the Québécois writer Catherine Mavrikakis's *A Cannibal and Melancholy Mourning*. The narrator hotly mourns all of these friends who have died of AIDS, all named Hervé. The narrator says she loves works that are tender and cruel, and that is what this is for me, a jeremiad, a beautiful complaint. The book is inspired by Hervé Guibert's autoportrait, *To the Friend*

Who Did Not Save My Life, fictionalizing his friend Michel Foucault's death from AIDS, which also documents Guibert's own diagnosis, like a French companion to *Close to the Knives*.

The interviewer asked me to talk about New Narrative, and I told him that it was an avant-garde queer mostly American literary scene circling around community, and especially memorializing friends and lovers who died of AIDS, refusing their disappearance. That in New Narrative, gossip is a political act, naming is a political act, a revolt against disappearance. I rattled off names of New Narrative writers: Bruce Boone, Dodie Bellamy, Kevin Killian, Kathy Acker, Gail Scott. The interviewer asked me if I thought there would ever be another movement where writers could be angry in force again, if there would be another crisis that would allow for a political literature.

I have thought about this question for a while now, and I think it connects to more than just writing—it's about art making; it's about a way of life that is opposed to a mainstream, homogenized success.

And I said to him that there is always something to be angry about, always something to rage against.

*

Can literature be a suicide note, a love letter, a manifesto, a complaint, can it be all of these things?

Can art be a way to trace not only disappearance, but our survival?

FRAGMENTS OF A LOST OBJECT

Meditations on the Photographs of Anne Collier

I am wondering what it means to collect.

*

I meditate upon the tender and witty memento mori of the photographer Anne Collier, who photographs her collections of books of photography, self-help tapes, other lost and melancholy objects.

*

"To collect photographs is to collect the world," Sontag writes in *On Photography*. A photograph in a book too, she notes, is an object to be collected.

*

Can you collect, I wonder, people too?

*

Anne Collier's image of Marilyn Monroe from Bert Stern's book *The Last Sitting*, from her Woman with a Camera series (the title teasing in its anonymity). Marilyn, in a moment of playfulness, poses with her black evening gloves and a Nikon camera suspended over her mouth, yet looks away, her eyes crinkling in a smile. The camera obscures but does not mask what we are really looking at—the face always so iconic, always a fact, so the camera performs a peekaboo, like the fan dance with the striped diaphanous scarf in those other Stern images. The camera isn't active, posed like it's actually looking back, taking pictures at the photographer capturing her. As if to show the joke: she is the beautiful image here; this is not her point of view.

*

So who is the woman with a camera? The woman with a camera is Anne Collier. Her gaze that is obsessive, sad, sensitive, witty. She's not just looking; she's looking at how others have looked (men, fellow photographers, all of us)—an affectionate and ironic distance, yet also with the intimacy of a collector, even, perhaps, a fan.

*

To look at this image of Marilyn Monroe is to mentally page through the rest of the book, with its morbid name—the fragility and pathos of those images—and then to linger on the biography, of Marilyn's deep unhappiness and struggle, which she would not survive. How this photo shoot, commissioned by *Vogue* in 1962, was part of a major publicity effort after she was fired from 20th Century Fox, a year after being institutionalized at Payne Whitney. How she would be dead of an overdose of barbiturates six weeks after she posed for these photographs over three boozy days in the Hotel Bel-Air. The heaviness of all of this, the tragedy behind closed doors, seeps into these photographs, giving them the weight of a historical memory. Memento mori, from the Latin for "Remember you will die."

*

And yet she performed such vitality. "You're beautiful!" Bert Stern remembers saying to Marilyn, upon meeting her. "What a nice thing to say," she replied, always rehearsed for her public. Upon seeing only accessories laid out on the bed, she quickly grasped his idea for the shoot, a series of nudes (not very high-concept). She was worried, initially, about revealing a surgical scar, but after consulting with her companion/hairdresser, she went for it. Champagne. Flirting. She became Marilyn (a movement she could do, how she could disappear into a crowd when not playing the persona, be a woman alone on a park bench). She transformed for the camera into the sex symbol. "Not bad for thirty-six," she said, once she came out of the bathroom in one of the sheer scarves.

*

There is no real intimacy to the nude, yet something was captured in these Bert Stern photographs, something, perhaps naked, unable to be replicated. He tried to replicate them, exactly, a few years ago, with Lindsay Lohan, but she possessed the tortured life but not enough of Marilyn's talent for vulnerability, her expressive and haunting face. Performances cannot be repeated, not exactly.

*

The red Xs of the contact sheets that Bert Stern published in the book, where Marilyn crossed out the images she disliked. The gesture that performs her disappearance. The cover of The Last Sitting is exactly this—Marilyn crossed out, Marilyn already a ghost, Marilyn's mouth open as if trying to say something.

*

Sontag speaks again: "Photographs state the innocence, the vulnerability of lives heading towards their own destruction, and this link between photograph and death haunts all photographs of people."

*

The camera is objective. And yet one desires to be inside, to enter a subjectivity hinted at in fragments. What does it mean to imagine another's life, the impossibility of accessing their first person? What does it mean to never escape one's image or mythic status, while still struggling with personhood?

*

A photograph to Sontag was also a fragment. This essay is composed of fragments. And by that I mean photographs.

*

Fragment: Marilyn reading James Joyce's *Ulysses* outdoors in the striped bathing suit. She often insisted on being photographed with a book (a desire to direct her publicity, perhaps, away from the image of the dumb blonde). This reminds me of the press photo of a young Louise Brooks, shiny in black-and-white, reading Kierkegaard on set.

*

Some English professor once called a method of skipping around reading *Ulysses* "the Marilyn Monroe method," as she confessed to not finishing it, and mostly enjoying Molly Bloom. The Marilyn Monroe method: I employ it too. I skip around. I flip. I drift.

*

I once wrote a series of failed monologues about screen sirens, imagining them as writers, as "difficult" women. Sirens—voices, ghosts, echoes. I imagined Marilyn as Molly Bloom, her fervent and ecstatic "I." Also: Veronica Lake, Vivien Leigh, Louise Brooks, Clara Bow, Judy Garland, really all the tragic ones. The ones who died young (tragic). The ones who died old (also tragic). The public selves constructed by the studio system, how this infected their private lives. A madness. To be alienated from oneself. Jean Harlow spoke of herself in the third person. "Jean Harlow was a figment of MGM's imagination."

*

Louise Brooks on Clara Bow, the It girl, an abstraction: "Off the screen she disappeared like an overexposed negative. The only thing she was was this image they had made for her."

*

What does it mean to share myths? Is it that these celebrities, these tortured women we have appropriated, tell us something about ourselves? A sort of projection. An overidentification. They met sad ends. They met lonely ends. They were alone in a room at the end.

*

I'm interested in difficult women, especially women who wanted to be artists, in their failures and fragilities, their uneasy communities with each other and refusals of kinship.

*

(This doesn't matter. This is not my self-portrait.)

*

The private "I" can search, tormented, as to one's contradictions. Marilyn's poetic fragments, written on hotel stationery, in unfinished diaries. In a letter to her therapist while at Payne Whitney: "Sometimes I wonder what the night time is for. It almost doesn't exist for me—." She was reading Freud's letters. She cried at his photograph, taken toward the end of his life. She thought he looked so sad.

*

I collect this fragment, this anecdote, and add it to my archives. My archives of loneliness and longing.

*

The isolation and identification between these figures. The stars were seen as repeats of each other. Gene Tierney on the ledge, recounting looking at Marilyn and Arthur Miller's apartment across the way. "It's Jean Harlow all over again," an exec at 20th Century said of Marilyn's screen test. Marilyn wanted to play Jean Harlow in a biopic. Her fascination with stars while growing up, in and out of foster homes. This is the narrative of the star system, of Hollywood. The desire to inhabit, to embody, someone else. That *Life* magazine photo spread of Marilyn dressed as Theda Bara, Clara Bow, Jean Harlow.

*

Can one's obsession be a form of autobiography?

*

Or one's gentle appropriation?

*

Louise Brooks: "Autobiography and biography are the greatest fictions."

*

To escape the self, in a portrait of another. That's acting. That's photography. That's perhaps writing too.

*

(What does it mean, then, to disappear?)

*

I count twenty-three neon Post-it notes marking the Bert Stern book in Anne Collier's photograph. I use the same type of Post-its, as a form of remembering—the moment of reading/looking, marking a return. The Post-its show the artist's touch and obsession—the hand, the eyes, two motifs reoccurring in her images.

*

The Post-its are lavender, lime, yellow, light pink, blue, hot pink. The coloring an affectionate nod to Warhol, as are her other Marilyn images, such as her side-by-side albums with Marilyn on the cover, and her witty single, diptych, and triptych of Marilyn heads against her gray studio floor, slightly fanned-out copies of Norman Mailer's book on Marilyn (another male auteur's appropriation of an actress).

*

An appropriation of Andy Warhol. A nod to his own act of appropriation—a meditation on media, celebrity. He created the Marilyn diptych weeks after her death, from a publicity photo from the 1953 film *Niagara*—a glamour shot, Marilyn in a sort of drag, in the lavish Marilyn mask. Set to Technicolor. Her publicity (not her private life).

*

Are there layers and levels of appropriation? Does it matter whether the feeling is of homage, or an inquiry, or that of ownership? Whether there's warmth and feeling, or detachment? I don't know. I think it matters.

*

Cindy Sherman dressing up, playing the anonymous starlet in her *Untitled Film Stills*. Anne Collier's photo of Cindy Sherman dressed in drag on the cover of a fashion magazine. Madonna dressing up as Marilyn in her most iconic stage, at the height of her stardom. Collier photographs a folded Steven Meisel poster of a nude and insouciant Madonna, cigarette in mouth, cupping her breast—the folds mimicking the grid of a Warhol. Gillian Wearing dressing up in drag as Warhol himself.

*

Kathy Acker wanted her punk texts that appropriated classic novels like *Don Quixote* and *Great Expectations* to be like a Sherrie Levine—like Levine's photographs of Walker Evans photographs. The litany of I's in Acker that are not her own. A way to inhabit, to wear a classic text from the inside. Unlike Anne Collier's appropriations, obviously inspired by the so-called Picture Generation, but kept at more of a witty gentle distance. Framed on a wall, in her own space, touched and manipulated by her hands.

*

So many eyes in Anne Collier's photographs. The witty take on *Un Chien Andalou*. The series of eyes in trays that reveal different photographic processes.

*

The left of Warhol's Marilyn diptych is colored, the right black-and-white, which Collier mimics in reverse in her Woman with a Camera diptych, of two framed press photographs of Faye Dunaway from a film Collier returns to, *Eyes of Laura Mars* (the title perhaps part of the obsession), a rather lurid film about a fashion photographer, played by Dunaway.

*

In the diptych, we are looking at two framed press photos hung on a wall, of Faye Dunaway posed with a Nikon camera, two different yet mirroring action shots. But she doesn't look like she is really using the camera, or at least the fingers posed on the camera are manicured impeccably, the hands staged almost awkwardly (the red nails of Cheryl Tiegs in another Woman with a Camera image, that same late-'70s glamour period Collier returns to, in this one it's even more evident that the camera is a prop). It is a playful image, but one that underscores the woman-as-image. But then in Anne Collier's layered doubling treatment of it, the subjectivity is given back, in some way. We can sense the heat of Collier's lens (her eyes, her camera) on the image, presumably shot by a male photographer, framed to show the ad copy, a series of male names. Collier's lens sensitive, aware, cognizant of technique as well as clichés, but also trained on the woman looking back. It is the traces of this—of the embodiment of the photographer, of what she is looking at—that gives these works such complexity.

*

And now I'm thinking of Warhol's later self-portraits, after Valerie Solanas shot him, after repeat surgeries, when he was paranoid that she would try again and obsessive about his own mortality. The self-portrait with his fright wig. The image, saturated in different pop colors but also the protection of camouflage, that looks more like a death mask (and he was to die nine months later from complications following gallbladder surgery).

*

What is the relationship of the death mask to self-portraiture? One cannot, literally, photograph one's own death mask. Marlene Dumas's painting of Marilyn pre-autopsy, *Dead Marilyn*.

*

Anne Collier appropriates another Warhol subject, Judy Garland, in her photograph of the book of consummate celebrity photographer Douglas Kirkland. The image that we see, marked off with a pink Post-it, is the 1961 still of an older Judy Garland crying—that intense, beautiful mask. Kirkland asked Garland to think of how sad her life had been, and she, the tortured ex-child-star and consummate performer, was able to cry on cue (although, like the self-conscious girl out of John Berger's *Ways of Seeing*, she has said she couldn't cry at her father's funeral). This is the Judy Garland who had survived collapses of her career and body and psyche, who had just the year before given that performance at Carnegie Hall, the glorious spectacle of her sobbing. She was to die eight years later at the age of forty-seven from an overdose of barbiturates.

*

The winds grow colder / Suddenly you're older, Judy belts out in "The Man That Got Away" from *A Star Is Born*, her Lady Lazarus performance after being fired by

MGM, that little pleased hiccupy laugh at the end of the song.

*

I too am somewhat of a fan, of a collector.

*

Measure the emotion, perhaps sentimentality, of not only Kirkland's photo but also Collier's appropriation (the intensity of the neon Post-it notes) with Warhol's diary entry about Judy Garland's funeral. More of a detached conceptualism, less of the adoration of a fan: "At the end of July I took Ondine and Candy up to the round-the-block line for Judy Garland at Frank Campbell's Funeral Home on 82nd and Madison. I wanted to tape-record them as they were waiting to go past the casket . . . I had it in my head that this would make a great play."

*

There is, to be sure, a fanaticism to being a fan. When thinking about Anne Collier's collecting, I go not only to Warhol but also to Joseph Cornell. He also used publicity shots—such as for his Penny Arcade Portrait of

Lauren Bacall. His shadow boxes that he made in his mother's basement in Flushing, Queens, are self-portraits in a way, the portrait of his obsessions, born of his collections. They work as well as devotional objects, shrines to his personal goddesses, actresses, ballerinas, his fellow poet-recluse Emily Dickinson.

*

Although Cornell was a hermit, he was also a walker of the city, where he would scavenge in used bookshops on Fourth Avenue, at five-and-dimes. Anne Collier searches in vintage stores, on eBay, for her record albums, books, photographs, from the '60s to the '70s.

*

The photographer and the collector are both obsessed with the past, says Sontag. She writes, "The collector becomes someone engaged in a pious work of salvage."

*

Joseph Cornell too was infatuated with Sontag, with her silver-striped, silver-tongued persona. He made her a collage as fan letter. Sontag, meditator on photography, also a celebrity, an image, the subject of so many famous portraits: by Mapplethorpe, Warhol, Peter Hujar, Diane

Arbus, and of course Annie Leibovitz, her later partner, the quintessential celebrity photographer.

*

I just got distracted reading online about Joseph Cornell's infatuation with a teenaged runaway waitress, named Joyce Hunter, who gave him his first kiss at the age of fifty-nine, and was later murdered. This the result of a search in which I asked Google: "Was Joseph Cornell kind of a stalker?"

*

The answer is, I think: Yes, but he was a sophisticated one.

*

There isn't, after all, a mutuality in obsession.

*

Collier's 2011 photograph named *Valerie*—a stack of different used editions of Valerie Solanas's *SCUM Manifesto*. The title and the repetition a nod to Warhol, again. By sheer force Valerie Solanas became a Warhol superstar, in her failed assassination attempt (terrible and macabre that the Garland song is still in my head, that crescendo—*The man that got away!*).

*

It was Valerie who was obsessed. The obsession was over a lost script, her play *Up Your Ass*, which she wanted Warhol to produce. She repeatedly returned to the Factory, demanding it back. Warhol paid her some money to act in two of his films. Lines she delivered with relish ("I gotta go beat my meat," she says in one). She also became convinced that Maurice Girodias of Olympia Press now owned all of her work. He had given her $500, apparently to write a novel based on her manifesto, which she was selling mimeographed on the streets when she met him (or maybe the payment was just to write a pornographic novel—there are different tellings). She wanted to be taken seriously as a writer.

*

It was Girodias actually who fictionalized the acronym as the "Society for Cutting Up Men." A cut-up. A collage.

*

That day she first went to the Chelsea Hotel to try to find Girodias. She showed up to the Factory dressed up in a black turtleneck sweater, raincoat, and, a rarity, makeup, as if she knew she might be photographed. (Warhol apparently said, "Doesn't Valerie look good!" upon seeing her.) When she finished shooting Warhol as well as the art critic Mario Amaya, she turned herself in to a traffic officer in Times Square.

*

"Read my manifesto and it'll tell you who I am," she apparently told him.

*

The connections between Warhol and Solanas have been made—both from working-class, Catholic backgrounds. The beginning of the *SCUM Manifesto*: "Life in this society being, at best, an utter bore." Warhol so attracted to boredom, to emptiness.

*

Collier's recent Questions series, her photographs of file folders containing pastel photocopies of questionnaires, worn and torn handouts.

CONNECTION

~How are things, events, or people connected to each other?

Pauline Oliveros's composition entitled *To Valerie Solanas and Marilyn Monroe in Recognition of Their Desperation.*

CONNECTION

Valerie felt the FBI was out to get her.

The FBI did watch Marilyn, recording her movements.

*

Valerie Solanas died broke and anonymous, at the age of fifty-two, in a welfare hotel in the Tenderloin district of San Francisco. One story has her still turning tricks, "slim and elegant" in a silver lamé dress. Another, maybe a parallel one, has her writing still, banging away at her outmoded typewriter, the landlord remembering her surrounded by pages and pages.

*

One of the voices of Sylvia Plath's radio play set in a maternity ward, *Three Women*, speaks to being the "heroine of the peripheral."

*

Anne Collier's photographs of tapes and albums, such as her 2008 photograph *Sylvia Plath*, the album propped against the wall on her studio floor, the title one can make out: *Sylvia Plath Reading Her Poetry*. The album cover an image of water and cliffs, at odds with the furious *Ariel* persona. Her clipped and draggy BBC radio narration. Sylvia Plath the opposite of self-help. And yet: the rushing sea.

*

Anne Collier's first photograph of her self-help tapes. These outmoded objects. Tapes framed inside their chalk-colored compartments, their casing operates as a sort of frame, photographed against a bone-white exterior. A sterility juxtaposed against the gentle irony of the sequence, its wordplay.

Introduction
Fear
Anger
Despair
Guilt
Hope
Joy
Love/Conclusion

That kills me, the last tape: Love/Conclusion. The promise of that. That by the time you get to the last tape, the listener will have rid herself of all bad feelings. Will have found Love—which will cancel out all negativity and destruction.

*

As if Love is ever a Conclusion.

*

But the way the casing has been warped, slightly cracked, suggests the use was not peaceful. The wear shows signs of vulnerability. And one thinks of the also yielding boundaries of the self. Its wear and tear. Its desire to heal from grief and loss, a desire so deep that it would cause someone to purchase these tapes. To use these tapes, perhaps. Then take an image of them.

*

I wonder looking at this heartbreaking yet subtle image— what is the monologue of Introduction? What is the monologue of Fear? What is the monologue of Anger (Valerie's, Sylvia's monologue)? And then I also wonder about the autobiography of those who used the tapes, their history. And yet it's so anonymous, and there is vulnerability I think to that anonymity. That is the pathos of self-help.

*

Another photograph, of a tape *Believe in Yourself*, half listened to: circa early '80s, probably. The purple capitalized type on the white tape, the illustrated purple stars.

*

The voice of these tapes—an interior voice we do not hear but can imagine—a repetition too, a mantra: to be okay, to be okay, to be okay.

*

When we are stuck, we look to other signs and systems to be okay in the world. To relieve the burdens of personhood.

*

For there is a sort of leveling off of the self in self-help. The first person is abstracted, universal. A litany of I's. A way of looking at the agonies of the self that is at once relieving and impersonal.

*

Anne Collier's First Person series. Nos. 1–4. Four large-scale photographs of pages of a book—a section called "Personality Profile Checklist." The statements of personality impersonal, contradictory, and thus quite deadpan. ("1. I am capable of giving orders. 2. I can easily show appreciation. 3. I am apologetic. 4. I can take care of myself.")

*

The lists Marilyn Monroe made for herself, to improve herself, to try to be happy. The affective labor of trying to survive. Lists, tapes, therapy, worksheets. The onus is on the individual.

*

Anne Collier's forms are not filled out. A photograph of a blank page entitled *Guilt* (presumably a journal entry to be filled out for a workbook?). Another photograph of a page entitled *What Do You Wish For?* (the magical repetition of "I WISH" then bracketed by an illustrated shooting star). *My Goals for One Year.*

*

Her unspooled tapes photographed against a white background, as if floating. The Anger tape unraveled first (the effect suggests dissipation, as does the memory of the gesture). It's a funny image. And yet there's some sort of quiet desperation or frustration to it. The unspooling too of Despair. Guilt. Problems. The feather-blue thread that comes out of the Hope tape.

*

A recognition of a suffering body. Or an annoyed body. (The tape is also a body.)

*

Another photograph entitled *Anger* actually refers to Kenneth Anger, of the lurid and gossipy *Hollywood Babylon* books (a fellow obsessive and collector), a photograph of two hands pressed into his handprints on the Walk of Fame.

*

The unspooled tapes almost form a shape of the emotion, something sculptural and figurative, this emotion that is supposed to be destructive, that the tape is serving to protect against. They are dancing and light when freed from their packaging.

*

And then her photographs of pirouettes of spools freed of their plastic bodies, their tangled figure eights. The kinetic sculptures of *Surviving Depression* or *Spiritual Warfare* or *The Unique and Mysterious Role of Hope*, almost Calder-like.

*

The dance posed between *Conflict, Criticism, and Anger*, one interprets something meaningful in this statement, how they are so bound up in each other.

*

Yet there's something to this. As opposed to focusing on the fiction of the integrated, instead to celebrate the beauty of the failures. The fragments of lost objects.

NEW YORK CITY, SUMMER 2013

On Kathy Acker

Ever since I moved here a few months ago I have been walking around looking for ghosts. Is it possible to mourn a city and time that I never knew? I walk around Alphabet City—how literary that sounds. Wild women like Cookie Mueller in the East Village. Nan Goldin's girls with their tears and pubic hair. Lydia Lunch ranting at the Pyramid Club. A young Kathy Acker walking around like a punk Edie Sedgwick bankrolled by Sol LeWitt. All the brilliant free spirits and so many of them are dead.

The week I got here I was asked to be on a panel on "literary bohemianism" with Katie Roiphe at McNally Jackson Bookstore. I said no.

The relationship of art to the market here feels psychotic. The conversations about writing here are conversations about publishing.

This city makes me feel psychotic.

I think of Kathy Acker's letters to Susan Sontag in *Great Expectations*, struggling over publicity, how to survive as an artist in this city. I want to hold a séance with Kathy Acker.

*

DEAR KATHY—
Who wants to be famous? Not me. But that is what is expected here. Visibility, brand, platform (gross gross gross). How can one artist survive here? And stay feral? How can art be political in society? (Rimbaud.)

DEAR KATHY—
I am experiencing career suicide ideation.

DEAR KATHY—
What defines the middlebrow to me is that it is absent of any anger, and by that I mean devoid of any politics. Why worry about the mainstream? Why can't we live and write in the margins? I know you write

that the margin is a way to be marginalized—that's why you hate "experimental." But I love that you hate. I love that you hate and that your works derive from such hate. I hate too.

DEAR KATHY—
But how to avoid feeling sold? Because I want to be successful, I want to be a success. What I would do sometimes for success, to not feel like a failure all the time, but success, I think, comes at a price, perhaps one's integrity. Did you feel too that American publishing is interested in success, not failure? When failure, I find, is so much more interesting.

DEAR KATHY—
Why can't I just be a boy genius?

DEAR KATHY—
I don't think New York City will ever love me. I don't think I'll ever love New York City.

*

All summer I kept on thinking of one of Jenny Holzer's texts: "IN A DREAM YOU SAW A WAY TO SURVIVE AND YOU WERE FULL OF JOY."

Kathy Acker lived in the same building as Holzer.

"Who can think about art in this miserable city?" In *The Adult Life of Toulouse Lautrec* Kathy made the painter a horny, ugly, alienated girl. New York City is Montmartre.

Still early on such an alive quality to the work. But this feels like a shift from the early plagiarism experiments. The "I" is and is not Kathy Acker. Raw and abject diary entries—yet filtered through art history and persona— destabilizing everything and giving it this A-effect.

"To survive in New York is to be a little like those hamsters on a wheel, the wheel turns faster and faster."

*

New York is exhausting and weird. I walk around Soho and look at all the rich bitches who are glacial in the extreme heat, wearing long sleeves. Either they are aliens or I am. What is it like to be so good-looking and gentrified?

Notes from a book proposal I try to write: "I want to write about feeling dirty and gross in public, as a woman and a writer, like a witch."

"I'm a total hideous monster. I'm too ugly to go out in the world . . . I'm extremely paranoid. I don't want to see anyone. I'm another Paris art failure. I'm not even anonymous. All I want is to constantly fuck someone I love who loves me."

The mannequin in the window at Catherine Malandrino wears a long red gown. Little specks of red paint splatter her white face. Like Carrie at the prom.

I've been making lists of how disgusting my body is. How chipped my black toenail polish. How filthy underneath my fingernails. The little toilet paper sculptures I pull out of my pubic hair.

Being groomed all the time feels impossible. I wonder if grooming is a desire to look simple and easy, to be easily read. I want a beautiful and perfect text like I want a beautiful and perfect body. I want to be seen as an intellectual, serious writer—but here I also want to be slim, young, fashionable. I walk around and suck in my stomach and worry over my yellow teeth. I buy expensive Acne white T-shirts like the models off duty wear, which on me just look like baggy white T-shirts. The day my book receives a (lukewarm) review in the *London Review of Books* I am obsessing over that, but also obsessing over pictures someone put on Facebook from the night before, at a friend's reading in Bushwick. My arms look so white and gross in a tank top, expensively shredded and newly procured. (My mother and her slim muscular arms, pointing out how flabby I am.) Ugh.

I go to a salon that all the other feminist writers on the Internet in NYC go to as well, run by a former Riot Grrrl who is also a feminist writer on the Internet. My models for haircuts are often writers I want to emulate—like Ann Quin's proud brunette head, or Gertrude Stein in Balmain, or elegant hollowed David Wojnarowicz, or austere rooster Samuel Beckett. These are often links I send to the photographer who needs to take my new author photo. I also send Robert Mapplethorpe photos of a young leonine Patti Smith, and then photos of an older warrior Patti Smith, and then the Peter Hujar of Susan Sontag reclining on the bed. I feel that's the image I want to project—fierce and striking, maybe scary. Intelligent and severe and masculine but also light pretty witty (cute). I am not sure which self I am anymore. I think probably I'm neither. I want to be ugly and bold, and then I want to be pretty and young.

I wanted to look like an alien, I told the person cutting my hair. Because that's how I've been feeling. The salon does not take my picture against the wall and put it up on their blog, like they do for another feminist on the Internet, who is something of a celebrity, a slim pretty blonde woman who knows how to pose for pictures. I have weird feelings about this other woman. She seems to encapsulate the New York literary scene for me—witty, bitchy, a popularity contest.

*

I have been sending little emails to myself thinking about this essay and this summer.

In the subject head: Identity Crisis.

In the body: "What does that mean?"

*

The summer before, I flew here to have my picture taken by a ladyblog. They said that I was One to Watch, and I wanted to be watched. I wore my black jersey Rick Owens. I got my hair newly shorn so I looked severe enough. The picture they chose to publish was me with my eyes closed. Otherwise you looked too intense, they said. At the party to celebrate the pictures I didn't know what to wear. So I bought a pink dress. Like a cotton pink day dress. Like the pink dress Villette buys.

Kathy Acker stares at us from those metallic pastel Grove Press covers, crimson-lipped and peroxide-butched.

I didn't want to smile in my author photo. Because for a while I always smiled, and this was something I wanted to resist.

Why isn't she smiling? My students asked me of Frida Kahlo. Kathy Acker was reading Frida Kahlo's biography on her deathbed.

I think of Kathy Acker like a gender-fucking Claude Cahun heroine. Muscled, tattooed, spiky-haired. Claude Cahun with a shaved head dyed green who freaks the fuck out of André Breton.

Her project one of hijacking literature, antagonizing memoir. As if there is a unified, coherent self. Kathy Acker manipulated this fiction. The author dies—*le petit mort.* Her personas the literary equivalent of Cindy Sherman's iconography. Can we contain all of these selves? Who is "I"? I can be the sum part of literature and history. I can insert myself inside.

The confessional as commodity, that is unleashed upon a coliseum. Kathy Acker torched this whole concept. She wrote the self, but she cast herself into the canon. She is writing the Young Girl far before Tiqqun. Except hers might be banal and entranced with her own image, she might have love stories, she might know her photo, but she is not a model citizen.

Kathy was image, fame whore—but then her texts are these wild experiments that fucked with all of this. The texts were the bombs. Acker refused to be invisible, yet she fragmented within her works. This is the compelling distinction. She presented a provocative, even scary image, refusing to be erased, but her texts enacted disappearance.

Her work was a manifesto for a writing and performance through and against shame and sickness and invisibility, gobbling up texts and vomiting them out, Mary Shelley as an eighteen-year-old girl terrorist. She satirized herself, made herself a grotesque. Her Janey Smith, her alter ego, exorcising her past girlhood.

*

The moment I turned the page to "Hello, I'm Erica Jong" in my *Essential Acker*, Elizabeth Wurtzel walked into the West Village Think Coffee with her black dog. Like a wraith out of this essay-in-progress. Her thin leopard scrunchie. The shiny face. The harsh blonde. She ate a sandwich wrapped in plastic and looked at her phone. And I realized she is one of my wounded monsters.

As am I. My nose dripping. I keep the crumpled dirty tissues in my purse like my mother did. The next day I am back at the same coffee shop, sobbing in public. Wounded over a recently ended friendship. Wondering too how I am going to survive as a writer, whether I'll ever be considered outside of the box of Angry Woman Writer.

A weariness to think that my life as a writer will be to just continue cannibalizing myself. I've begun to question myself—what is self-promotion and what is inquiry, connecting the self to something larger? The lines for me have become blurred.

I write in my notebook: "Elizabeth Wurtzel vs. Kathy Acker?"

The difference is maybe multiplicity. A refusal to commodify a coherent self. Or ugliness. I mean, I don't know.

*

That a good girl named Karen Lehmann could shed her skin and become Kathy Acker (Acker her married name). Could shed that skin again and dissolve and fragment.

She is Karen or Kathy like I am a Katie or a Kate. We have good-girl names.

All the Karen Lehmanns I google.
Karen Lehmann is a wedding photographer in North Carolina.
Karen Lehmann is a librarian in Iowa.
Karen Lehmann is a real estate agent in Florida.
Karen Lehmann is an ear, nose, and throat surgeon in South Africa.

One Karen Lehmann from NYC married a lawyer, announced in the *NYT* wedding section.

I realize that my writing is about conjuring up and murdering the girl I was and have allowed myself to become, a tender horror. I channeled my past self into all of these toxic girls . . . An "I" that is not only about my past but also about my present self, still gagging on all of my contradictions. Marguerite Duras with her ravaged face and whisky calling back to the girl she was. Clarice Lispector writing her girl in the markets at São Paulo while dying of cancer. "Am I a monster or is this what it means to be a person?"

Kathy Acker's girls are fools (dogs) for love, forced into humiliating roles within capitalism. Lousy, mindless salesgirls, strippers, daughters in love with fathers. They are not empowered. But she is not (just) (directly) documenting masochism or abjection or a double bind, I don't think. This is not transcription. It's alienation. It's depersonalizing the concept of confessionalism and the self. It doesn't offer itself up to be easily consumed.

Romance narratives that colonize our brains she made into campy soap opera. Like the opening of *Blood and Guts in High School*, my first introduction to Acker—Janey Smith in love with her father. Later Janey is the dog trailing after a cruel Genet. Fucking the ambivalent father. Of

Blood and Guts she said, "I wanted to take the patriarchy and kill the father on every level."

The contemporary consciousness is not a stream. It is jarring, fictive, evasive, colonized by other fictions and narratives.

I love the artists who portray the girl as a potential terrorist but who view this skeptically, from a loving yet sometimes satirical distance, understand her indoctrination too into passivity, her ambivalent libertinism—Elfriede Jelinek, Vera Chytilová, Marguerite Duras, Kathy Acker. Rimbaud said he wanted to make himself the experiment and experience itself the poison.

Kathy Acker is not insincere—sometimes she taps into a vein of such deep feeling.

She's conceptual but not bloodless, totally impure.

*

Anne Carson said of Francis Bacon that with his paintings, his portraits of viscera and horror, he removed a boundary. This is what Kathy Acker did too. She removed a boundary.

Lately I have been thinking of writing as a visitation. Genet nailing his criminals to the wall. Kathy in a form of drag.

When one gets crazy and risky, perhaps beautiful things can happen. Can one push against an internalized conservatism?

"It's necessary to go to as many extremes as possible."

*

In an interview with Sylvère Lotringer (Kathy Acker's longtime lover), Julia Kristeva speaks of Céline's "opera of the flood," how it takes from an aesthetic based on the borderline, the oozy types who go back and forth from publicity to withdrawal.

Since moving here I have taken to wearing too much makeup. Old-lady makeup. Penciled red lips, Chanel red, penciled-in brows, black eyeliner.

Sometimes I feel skinless, raw. Like I don't have a face. How can I be sure that I have any coherence unless I outline it?

*

This is how I've figured out the Internet. Once in a while when I'm feeling particularly fragile I'll binge on googling myself. But to practice self-care I'll avoid combinations like my name and "I hate," things like that.

Then I go on Twitter and Facebook approximately five hundred times until I feel sick and crazy.

When I binge online, I feel paranoid, fearful, oozy, weird, itchy, unhealthy, unsafe, stressed.

"I'm a failure. This is a failure all I'm craving is my own disintegration . . ."

This psychosis triggered on or by the Internet, our repository of confessions.

Fernando Pessoa's heteronyms and Kathy Acker's personas the contemporary condition of our fragmentation.

I would have loved to have witnessed Kathy Acker terrorize the Internet.

*

Would a commercial press take a chance on Kathy Acker's writing now? I think they would say too unfinished, violent, porny, queer, risky, litigious. They would say "too unreadable." "This is not what the reader wants." And Kathy responds: "I could give a fuck about what the reader wants." Her work is not based in continuous character or narrative.

The promise of success and being self-congratulatory is so seductive here—to turn in bourgeois narratives that prey on identification. Thomas Bernhard, the Great Viennese Hater, flips this and makes his characters total frauds. Kathy Acker, our Great American Hater, makes them fictions.

There needs to be a word, I've realized, for the parasitism of middlebrow art and literature that steals from interesting and radical art but in the process strips it of its ferality, its political urgency, its queerness, its threat. (Sarah Schulman uses the term "gentrified," also connecting it to Acker.)

DEAR KATHY—
How can I plot to throw a bomb in the face of my possible success, which I do not want?

Kathy antagonized the commercial mind-set. And she is still so often misread, mischaracterized. Seen as a trick or stylistic pyrotechnics that can be easily imitated. That is not to say her works are not readable, which is often what I'm told. Her works are not *easy*. Because they are not meant to be easily consumed or simply titillating. None of her books need to be finished. They deal with what Sianne Ngai has called "ugly feelings." Her work engages in tedium, annoyance, revulsion, titillation, confusion, similar to the "selective inattention" of witnessing avant-garde theater.

There is no room for decorum within a Kathy Acker text. She takes the brutal flood of sex and violence in Guyotat and further dismays it—not only copies it, destabilizing the reader, a fuck funhouse where she jerks you around after jerking you off. Her porn texts are too prickly to jack off to without feeling the threat of castration.

"I want to say 'fuck, shit, prick.' That's my way of talking, that's my way of saying 'I hate you.'"

A great artist is not meant to be consumed, but to devour.

This work that is like a tremendous terrorism against the body of white male literature. Writing against and appropriating and inserting herself into Great Male Texts. Taking on the role of the hysteric, the mimic, like Irigaray. Acker is Pip in *Great Expectations*. She is Don Quixote the knight having an abortion, trying to awaken as a great artist. At the opening of *Don Quixote* the green paper of the hospital gown turns into writing paper. Writing the body. Writing sickness. Janey Smith walking around with pelvic inflammatory disease.

DEAR KATHY—

You and David W. argue for the political necessity of writing about the sick body, to counteract silencing. Like David W. you contracted a diseased society as well. Your rants against the government, against war and hypocrisy. Anyone that depoliticizes you has essentially misread you.

DEAR KATHY—

I know I should wait until I'm like sixty to reject and radicalize my youth in writing, but what if I never make it to then? That's what I keep on thinking. It feels inevitable to me, to die of cancer of the lady parts. I think of your work's urgency. How you just kept on writing books. You knew you were finished when you got bored. These games you played. I think of all of them as one book, punctuated by covers bearing your face.

DEAR KATHY—

David W. died and you died and one needs to make work of great risk and threat and vulnerability just as one needs to expose oneself to great risk and threat and vulnerability because we will die. Otherwise you will die. But you left behind a body of work—such a grotesque beautiful glittering body. An infuriating body, a provocative body. A body that raged.

DEAR KATHY—

I dream of you and you are devouring. I mix you up with my mother in my mind. My mother who died of cancer. Your mother's suicide. I think of you like my mother, mysterious and hard-nailed, evading with lies and myths. You are as slippery as she was.

DEAR KATHY—

You would tell your writing students to write about having sex with their weirdest family member. I feel with you something Oedipal edible. A devouring. The intimacy I feel for you, that would not have been reciprocated in real life. But it is an intimacy, a connection, that I need desperately.

DEAR KATHY—

Everyone wants to tell me you didn't get along with other women writers. I don't need other people to tell me this. I love Dodie Bellamy's description in her essay on your clothes—about how you weren't friends but were suspended in a mutual admiration and respect, on her side love—how when she once passed you at a party or reading she had a moment of true knowledge that intimacy would be impossible. That you would devour each other.

DEAR KATHY—
I want to write book after book of repulsive women.

DEAR KATHY—
Women writers I now see and admire as fellow monsters, prickly, wounded, devouring, but I feel I can't get too close. I've wanted them to mentor me. It's impossible, except on the page. They now want me to mother them. Yet I am an unfit mother. I am a barren womb. Don't approach me and say you want to read me—which is telling me you want to love me—I will devour you, I will fill your life with so many words until you have none.

DEAR KATHY—
Was it the same for you?

DEAR KATHY—
Maybe this is because we are denied much crucial space in the culture. But you took up space. You never asked for permission.

DEAR KATHY—

The prickliness I feel for my peers, a paranoia. I want their respect more than anything. You craved community too but always felt like an outsider.

DEAR KATHY—

Kathy, it's reviews by other women that have hurt the most. I am my texts. My texts are not feminist enough, too feminist, too sickly, too passive, too in love with fashion, etc.

DEAR KATHY—

I have begun taking pictures of old ladies on my iPhone. It's making me love New York. My true jouissance would be getting inside the closet of Manhattan ladies with their art bobs who bought '80s Comme des Garçons. I think of you in your Gaultier with sweat stains. I look at pictures online of Michèle Lamy, Rick Owens's wife and muse. Her psychotic crone gorgeousness. The black eyeliner she draws on her forehead to center herself. I love decadent crones, psychotic crones, gorgeous crones who don't give a fuck. That's who I wish to be.

DEAR KATHY—

I'm glad I haven't met you, in a way. I can read your texts as sustenance, as encouragement. I don't feel weird or crazy you won't blurb my book, or act diva-like with me, or didn't want to read with me. I'm sure you were sometimes dreadful, sometimes a monster, generous, complex. But I don't have to feel bitter or wounded or ignored—I can just feel fully your work and influence. I can love you completely.

ONE CAN BE DUMB AND UNHAPPY AT EXACTLY THE SAME TIME

On Failure, the Depressed Muse, and Barbara Loden's Wanda

Fourth of July, 100 degrees outside. I am an insect trapped in sticky, humid amber. I keep on shifting the thermostat—74, 73, 72. I have been home alone for weeks at our cottage in the small hippie town of Carrboro, North Carolina. My partner, a rare books librarian, is off to Oxford on a fellowship to study Tudor-era books. We flew to Europe together, a small holiday before—Paris, Amsterdam, Antwerp. Now I'm home. I am supposed to write, of course. I am always supposed to write. Some sort of misery, being in between projects. Feeling stuck.

I leave the house once a day to take our terrier on a walk. It is a sauna outside and the puppy rebels, lies down stubborn on the grass. His coat a magnet for the sun—all black except for the darling silver mohawk, enhanced at my request by the groomer. I occasionally carry him home, him prone like an endangered maiden. Sometimes I try to drag him, an impotent gesture. Not the best idea to name your puppy Genet, especially in the South. I tell people he's named after a French anarchist.

The same mile loop around the leafy neighborhood. When I walk, I feel like Duras's housewife Lol Stein, who is attempting through her circumambulations to get back to her girlhood. Lately I feel like I am sleepwalking through a large strange space that's something like grief. I have to remember that I'm still jet-lagged. A slowness to everything. A particular sense of drift.

To walk the dog I dress in costume—a way to alleviate the heat and perhaps the dullness. Sweaty short-shorts and a large floppy fedora and high-heeled sandals, like a thirtysomething zaftig version of the girl in Duras's *The Lover*. The narrator, a writer now, remembering the passivity and dumbness of her youth. Something about the meditative quality of the silence here also makes me feel like a Duras heroine.

Today we have to cross a parade of muscled, fervent marathoners. Genet and I watch them for a time, admiring their bodies' velocity. Finally I pick the dog up and, breathing apologies, we shuffle through the throng.

*

When I think about what I want this essay to be, I think about walking through an open space. Maybe when walking, the body is essaying. A wandering, a wondering. An essay attempts, in the tradition of Montaigne. The idea of an essay as an attempt reveals the possibility, perhaps the pull, of its failure. The slowness of all of this.

When walking in my neighborhood in the sticky heat, clomping carefully in my wooden heels, trying to think through things, I am aware of myself as an absurd yet tentative figure in the landscape. Lol Stein in a trance. The somnambulist Robin Vote in Djuna Barnes's *Nightwood*.

The actress Barbara Loden trudging up the hill of black coal in her 1970 film *Wanda*, playing the eponymous Scranton housewife who has abandoned her family, who has been set adrift, who eventually finds herself involved in a botched bank robbery.

A figure in white, like a ghost, still haunting a barren landscape where she is no longer functional, making her way almost glacially through rich black. It is meditative, this monotony. A spectral, Sisyphean scene.

Wanda is a film about an impoverished woman who cannot escape the stagnant circle her life has become. Shot in cinéma vérité style and mostly improvised, it is the only film that the actress and wife of the director Elia Kazan made.

This was her attempt, her meditation—on failure, on isolation, on being trapped.

The opening scene. Close-up on a baby screeching in a dirty diaper. Wanda has walked away from being a mother and wife, yet she is still cloistered in a squalling domestic space, crashing at her sister's house. She is the ghost shrouding herself under sheets on the couch, hungover, hiding.

Barbara Loden channeling a past of muted poverty for her character, growing up bewildered and stuck in a mountain town of North Carolina, living with her fundamentalist grandparents. She remembered hiding behind the kitchen stove, wondering who she was, wondering what she was doing there. This is why Elia Kazan told her he cast her as the Marilyn Monroe stand-in for the stage version of Arthur Miller's *After the Fall*. He cast her because he said that she and Marilyn were both orphans. She was his mistress for years before he married her. Marilyn Monroe also at one time Kazan's mistress. A mirroring.

I keep on writing about Barbara Loden. This is not the first time I've attempted to write about her. I can't seem to figure her out.

To circle: an obsession. Trying to decipher, to imagine past fates.

*

At midnight I stand outside on the back patio in only a tank top and underwear, staring out at the height of the pine trees. I watch Genet prowl and bark at the deer hiding in the small wooded area behind our fence. The ways in which jet lag mimics depression. I think: Yes, perhaps I am losing my mind. Like I can see this calmly, objectively. Too much isolation. When your voice sounds strange, calling out in the distance.

I have to remind myself my body is still weak. After two lovely days strolling around Paris with John, I became sick in Amsterdam with a throat infection. For days I lay on the blue velvet sofa of the Airbnb apartment in the Jordaan district, drifting in and out of feverish sleep, listening to the roars of drunk Russian men on booze cruises in the canal, too weak to even walk around except to go to a tourist doctor with a haphazard and somewhat seedy office who wrote me a script for a tri-pak of antibiotics.

I canceled the rest of my trip. I was supposed to go to Berlin and Paris by myself, and then meet John up in London for the weekend. The plan is to visit him again in July.

The antibiotics acted fast, like a shot. By the flight home I was feeling more alive, yet somehow altered. I returned to the green stickiness of North Carolina alone.

So intensely nostalgic, that throat infection. I used to get them all the time. Being a toxic girl in my twenties and showing boys at bars my massive pus pockets in the back of my throat, like a parlor trick, while I smoked menthols and jammed popsicles down my throat as my medicine. Remembering what it was like to be unsafe and unhygienic and uninsured, almost radiantly fucked up.

Thinking of the ways nostalgia can also be a disease.

*

I always confuse Barbara Loden with the character she plays in her film *Wanda*, and then those two figures with this girl I once lived with in Chicago. The girl I knew was ten years older, so the last time I knew her, she would have been thirty-five, the age that I'm going to be this year. I think a lot about her. Like Barbara Loden, she's someone I'm always trying to figure out.

I met this girl while waiting lunch tables one summer at a bourgeois Italian café in Bucktown—the café tried on the surface to be old-world authentic with its grappa selection and gelato case but was really fake, with its faux-fresco mural of smiling waving people. She worked as a barista, expertly making espresso drinks. I was in an oozy dumb period then—I had an older musician boy-friend, we'd get drunk at bars. I worked in a bookstore as well, and would sit and read Kathy Acker at the register and refuse to shelve books. I wore a lot of short dresses then. I remember this one beige and backless cotton dress with red piping and a white slip underneath that I tied in back, like a subversion of an apron. I wore the dress with red platform heels that I paired with everything, that got all scratched up and white in the rubber wedge. My best friend, an art student and hostess at the local pan-Asian place, had those shoes, and I coveted them, and then got my own.

I was depressed, quite often. Sometimes I would sit in my room and scribble in my journal. But most of the time I just tried not to think about anything too seriously. I remember my youth as a period of vague incoherence and often intense emotional pain that I did not know how to voice. My unhappiness did not yet have a political context.

*

On one level I think my connection between this girl I used to know and Barbara Loden is the uncanny simi-larity of their presences—the fine blonde hair, the little fox face, the girlish frame, the soft, nasally voice. As with Barbara Loden's Wanda, there was something so tragic and passive about my friend, I always thought. How she would tiptoe around the apartment, landing softly on the balls of her feet like a ballet dancer. Like she didn't want to be heard. Like she didn't want to take up too much space.

She had an old-fashioned, mellifluous name, like an expected name change for a player in the MGM factory, an even more old-fashioned nickname. I guess I'll have to call her something. I'll call her Veronica, Ronnie for short, as she did have a Veronica Lake quality to her, especially when she would curl her long feathery blonde hair around her to hide within. Except she was closer to the later Veronica Lake, who became a drifter, working as a barmaid at the Martha Washington Hotel in New York City once her movie career was ruined. God. The story of Veronica Lake is so sad. Like Frances Farmer, who also went from movie star to a life adrift and subservient and perpetually boozy, folding towels in a Seattle hotel. Veronica Lake's multiple arrests for public drunkenness, staying at seedy hotels, madly in love with a merchant seaman, finally a shut-in in Hollywood, Florida (yes), fearful of being stalked by the FBI.

I'd like to write a book that's like Shulamith Firestone's *Airless Spaces*, but about Hollywood stars who became hermits who refused to leave the house, having lost their looks and career and most often money, spiraling, shuttled in and out of institutions, trying to escape from their public and former selves, uncertain of their identities, sometimes paralyzed with rage. Clara Bow, Louise Brooks, Gene Tierney, Veronica Lake, Frances Farmer, Vivien Leigh.

As I am writing this, Shulamith Firestone has just been reported dead. She withdrew from public life after *The Dialectic of Sex*, which was written in her twenties. And then years later this drifting series of reminiscences, published on Semiotext(e)'s Native Agents, that reminds me of Anna Kavan's diaristic *Asylum Piece*. In *Airless Spaces* Firestone draws from her own experiences being institutionalized to write vignettes of those she encountered who were forgotten by the system, given a diet of pills to control their alienation and violence. In the work the language comes with difficulty—she writes of a character who was reading Dante fluently before being institutionalized, who afterwards couldn't even flip through magazines. And yet she summons up scenes of this stuck, slow circle of hell. Guards pulling a naked woman into the shower. Hydrotherapy. Bloated bodies. Anorexic bodies. Abject bodies.

The narrator in *Airless Spaces* often meditates on losing her looks in the hospital. The back of the small blue book is haunting—Firestone's visage, looking out bespectacled and eagle-like, her trademark long dark hair almost brutally shorn.

Firestone lived to sixty-seven—an old age actually for such a life, of poverty, suffering, isolation, decades in and out of institutions.

*

After only a few months of our working together, Ronnie let me move in with her when I decided to move out of the apartment I was living in with another girl. My friendships with girls back then were like tortured, passionate love affairs, always ending badly and with a spectacle of acrimony. A series of falling out, of falling in, of quick kinships. Then I moved in with my boyfriend, began to work as a writer and an editor, broke up with my boyfriend, went to grad school for a time. Then Ronnie and I didn't see each other for a while. I moved home when my mother got sick, commuted to the city to work.

When my mother died, we bumped into each other on Damen Avenue, both of us at ends of situations, me having given up my lease in that doll's studio in Lincoln Square to move home, first to take care of my mother and then to tend to my widowed father. She told me horror stories of her roommates, messy strangers in Logan Square, she perennially prickled and flustered. We spontaneously decided to move in together again. I liked the idea of living with someone who knew me. After my mother died, I went through a period of not wanting to be alone for long periods of time. I wonder if I've gone out of that period.

At least with Ronnie I knew what I was getting into. In some ways we were intimates. In other ways we were strangers. I was always so tentative with her, me tiptoeing in a way as well, never really pushing her or questioning her. She would just sometimes snap at you. Her quick turns.

During the inevitable moving out, when Ronnie decided to go live with the girl with the red shoes, which I saw as an absolute betrayal, we each yelled at the top of our lungs that the other needed help. It was true. We both did need help. My parents paid for my therapy for a while after college, but then cut me off. Ronnie tried to get help several times, standing in an eternal line at a public health center, but without insurance, it was basically impossible, or at least it seemed so, at the time.

The ambivalence toward others in *Airless Spaces*. Sometimes having a roommate feels like living in a mental ward. Does the outside mirror the inside or reverse?

When my mother was put in the psychiatric ward, despite stage-four lung cancer, I would visit her there every
day. Or whenever I could. Whenever I could force myself.
My father and I would sit outside of her room in hard-
backed chairs. My brother, sister, sometimes too. She was
put in the ward with the old people. Remembering how
they would force her to sit in the public area, an exhausted
shaven baby, skinny and brown, her hospital gown gaping
open, while the demented patients drank juice and played
games.

*

The idea for *Wanda* came from a newspaper clipping of
a woman in England convicted of being an accomplice
in a bank robbery. She thanked the judge when he sen-
tenced her for twenty years. "That's what struck me:
Why would this girl feel glad to be put away?" Loden
said in an interview.

At the beginning of the film, Wanda is late for her divorce hearing, having to go to the mines in her outfit of
white jeans and hair curlers in order to borrow money
for the bus from an elderly worker who might be her
father. Her estranged husband is already at court with
their crying children and the new woman, a substitute
nursemaid.

She has nothing to say as a rejoinder to her husband, who is speaking of her uselessness as she wanders into the courtroom. Nothing to say to the judge. "Your husband says you've deserted him and the children. What do you have to say about it?" Throughout the film she often looks like she's in trouble, aware that she's being disciplined, but she lacks language. She is muted. "Nothing," she says, shrugging. Not with attitude. More— numbness.

*

For years I did not know what happened to Ronnie. A few times I spied her on the streets from afar when I still lived in Chicago. I recognized her by her dainty gait. I thought perhaps she could have been a suicide. Or someone who just faded out, got lost in the system, stuck eternally in some dead-end situation. But I wonder if she thought that of me as well. I mean, maybe she knew I transcended things, became an editor, a writer, formed a lasting relationship. But perhaps she always suspected I would switch back, go back to my real fate of fucking up and failure. Maybe that's why I write. I'm sure this has something to do with why I publish. To announce to myself, as well as to the drifts of former intimates, that I am still alive. The beat of the heart. Like Esther Greenwood attending her alter ego's funeral in *The Bell Jar*. I am. I am. I am.

The last section of *Airless Spaces* is entitled "Suicides I Have Known."

That other girl I lived with the time before, the psychology major, did kill herself—I attended her Irish-Catholic wake on the South Side years later, even though we had not spoken for years, her bloated in the casket and wearing a flowery dress she never would have worn in real life. In many ways she was more like Wanda than the girl I mix up in my head with Wanda. But I've already written about this other girl before. I don't mean to now. I've already summoned her up.

And yet I've summoned up Ronnie before, for my antiheroine Ruth in *Green Girl*. Once I became a writer, Ronnie became a belated muse for me, of a certain model of alienation. I mythologized Ronnie, like Barbara Loden did with Wanda. Although Ruth was also a young Catherine Deneuve, and also the silent cool blonde girl who lived downstairs while I was writing the book. And she was me of course. They're always me of course.

One can become a suicide by being forgotten.

Something about witness. *Airless Spaces* is dedicated to "Lourdes Cintron—as promised in the hospital."

Eventually, once I read Jean Rhys, I began to think of Ronnie as a character out of one of her novels, not one of her impressionable ingénues but one of her older women, numbed out, who tries to suppress her rage in public, who is frozen by past affairs. Like Sasha Jensen in *Good Morning, Midnight*.

I never got the whole story of her life before she knew me. I got it in fragmented reminiscences. Ronnie hoarded past memories, especially the bitter ones. The repetition of certain names. I knew the name of the boy she should have married. I perennially heard the name of the boy who almost destroyed her.

In her twenties Ronnie lived in Detroit, and she would always recall those times with such intense nostalgia. I find myself doing this now with the Wicker Park neighborhood of Chicago, which is where I lived with Ronnie and with many others, knocking around there for a decade. Remembering when you couldn't catch a cab in the neighborhood, why would you, you'd never be able to afford a cab, this before the valet parking appeared and everyone I knew had to move.

Remembering that time when your city had possibility, had space, before all the others moved in, before we all moved out, which really is a stand-in for when we had unrealized possibility, the drifting period of our youth.

(Of course we were also the others who moved in—those who must move out are erased.)

*

Afternoons I sit outside on the front porch, Genet curled into me on one of the chairs. To sit and watch and be slow in the heat feels distinctly southern. Sometimes, although not often, I am able to read, and it's wonderful, to be able to sink into something. I eat too-expensive cherries and reread Mary Gaitskill's *Bad Behavior*, the reddened tips of my fingers turning the pages. Her dingy world of fuckups trying to escape their stuckness through desperate contact with other people. Her characters caught in absolute tedium. They desire to lay waste to their days. Like the vagabonds in Jim Jarmusch's *Stranger Than Paradise* staring at a procession of images on the television.

*

Ronnie and I both worked strings of temporary jobs where we were always quitting or being fired. A few gigs at a time. Mine were mostly in restaurants. Months before I got the café job I had worked at the Hollywood, a twenty-four-hour diner just down the street on North Avenue, a job I suddenly walked away from, during a paralyzingly slow afternoon shift. This was a semiregular performance for me. Just walking out. Some quick glimpse of freedom—although of course I'd always have to find a job that was more of the same.

It was called the Hollywood, yet there was nothing glamorous about it—the owner, an enterprising Greek man, short and squat with a glint in his eye, had commissioned an appropriately themed wall painting, Marilyn Monroe, Elvis, James Dean, etc. The oldies station played all the time. We wore turquoise-green polos with purple collars that said the name of the restaurant in script on the back. I was one of the only girls working there—except the niece of the manager, a beautiful girl who trained pit bulls, who later got into a car crash that fucked her face up and made her a bit off afterwards, or so I heard. The manager was a Canadian guy who would whisper to me about his life as an agent for the CIA. Whenever I came in, he would tell me stories about dressing in drag or jumping out of airplanes—I'm not sure if he thought I believed him, or if he believed himself. He gave me two pieces of advice that I remember to this day: always buy good shoes and premium orange juice.

To work at the diner I would dress in a costume as well—a variety of bandannas I'd tie my hair back with, dark red lipstick that clashed with the green and purple. We served hipster kids coming in from the bars, cops, workers from the S/M club, the strip club, the tattoo parlor, families who spoke all different languages, construction workers, yuppies, the sex workers who walked up and down North Avenue and hung out at the Home Depot. Sometimes their pimps. The regulars would tell us their stories. When I did the overnight shift, I'd take herbal Ecstasy and drown it in a liter of Mountain Dew from the gas station across the street. I'd sleep the entire next day to recover.

Ronnie had worked as a house cleaner, as a companion to a female shut-in, in a factory, in telemarketing, at shitty office temp jobs. She worked as a cigarette girl for a marketing company for Camel when I knew her. They hired cute girls to go to assigned bars when they were packed and give out free packs of cigarettes, for giving your information. That was one of the regular things she did— even when she didn't have anything else going on, she'd go to work at 11 PM. She would return home, drained. It would be difficult to wake up the next day if she had an earlier shift somewhere else. So sometimes she didn't. She'd often call in sick to her jobs when she just couldn't force herself to go.

Capitalism made us sick. Forced us into humiliating roles.

*

At the beginning of the film, Wanda goes to the factory where she recently worked, her hair curlers and shuffling gait in counterpoint to the brisk models of efficiency making dresses. She asks tremulously about her pay for the last week. She also asks for more work. "I'm sorry, my dear," the piggy boss man condescends to her. "You're too slow in our operation, and we can't use you." Still, she thanks him, haltingly.

That flashback scene in Jean Rhys's *Good Morning, Midnight*, where Sasha Jensen remembers being fired at the atelier by the boss who tests her on how well she knows German. But in the novel we get the interior monologue of Sasha's impotent fury, her fury at herself for her passive reaction in the moment, that she still has to go through the motions to try to please this man, a feat that she knows is impossible. In the film we only get Wanda's blank face, her rote expression of gratitude that is more a stand-in for numbness.

The factory girls in *The House of Mirth*. Lily Bart's vague feelings of philanthropy toward these down-and-out girls with pretty faces. She gives them money, money that slips through her hands. Later in the novel, when due to scandal her chance of a good marriage has slipped away, her well-meaning friends set her up an apprenticeship at a millinery. They imagine her owning a small shop making hats for posh clientele. Yet she is too slow. Her fingers too untrained. She is told to undo simple tasks by the woman looking over her. She cannot exist, working like this, under these conditions.

*

Ronnie and I both got unceremoniously fired from the Italian café soon after I moved in with her in her one-bedroom apartment, in that dead-end area near the Kmart and the Blockbuster off the highway (the Blockbuster long ago bulldozed to make room for a luxury car dealership), me dragging my dirty futon mattress into her tiny hole of an extra room. We were both fired for the usual bullshit reasons, but really it was because it was the end of the summer and they didn't need the extra help anymore. She was laid off the day before and then I was the next day, showing up to work, finding my time card not in its slot. So then you knew you had to go see the manager. How humiliating it was to have piggish bosses smirk at you, to have to listen to their assaults on your character, to feel absolutely powerless. They lectured you on how to live your life, as if they knew. As if they had any fucking idea.

I can still see Ronnie sitting cross-legged on her grandmother's brocade sofa when I came home after being fired from the café, eating a bowl of popcorn, watching a film on the small TV on the floor, a Hal Hartley film she'd watch over and over, *Henry Fool*. It was the only film she owned. When I told her, she threw her head back and laughed, a throaty, acidic peal that I rejoiced in hearing, probably because it was so rare. For other times she was so moody, silent, as was I, us circling each other. It was one of those moments. Of complete fuck, what are we going to do now?

In our own ways we were used to stretches of unemployment while waiting to find something, of even waiting then for weeks until we got our first paycheck. That's why I preferred to work for tips. We were both intimate with payday loans. We weren't getting help. Both of us had strained relationships with our families. We got by on three dollars a day. Sometimes we would eat cereal all day. I can see us, sitting on the stoop in the second place we lived together, on Damen, eating Lucky Charms out of a box. The addicts that loitered outside. The three yippy little dogs who lived upstairs. We would dream murderous thoughts about them. Ronnie would take a broom and bang on the ceiling. I guess we both cracked. Maybe we didn't break up with each other. We broke up with that place.

*

Although I knew that this would not be my certain fate. I felt sure in some way I could escape from it. I was still quite young when I knew Ronnie, in my early twenties. Now I'm the same age she was when I last knew her. Yet I am not broke anymore. Not desperate. My spouse with his academic library post. In most places we've lived I had regular gigs teaching. My bachelor uncle, my father's identical twin, left me a small inheritance two years ago when he died, rather agonizingly, of liver cancer. Like Virginia Woolf's aunt. Yet I need to find work soon. I cannot find teaching work, women and gender studies curriculums being slashed in North Carolina. So still circling, circling around. Going back to apply to "girl" jobs.

Yesterday I donned my new black-and-gold silk dress, quite ladylike at the knees, and my sandaled heels, in order to go for a job interview at Duke University for a part-time administrative assistant position for a famous professor in the literature department. The office dowagers spoke about him in hushed tones, as they did all of their scholars (I figured out it was the Chilean writer Ariel Dorfman). I wonder what it would be like to be treated with such respect. The woman in charge eyed my four-inch heels as I clomped up the stairs, in the un-air-conditioned hallway.

I didn't get the position. I didn't even get called back for a second interview. There is a sort of voluptuousness, I think, about almost permanently occupying this realm of failure.

The gnawingness of being perennially unemployed. The occasional seizure of despair. Especially when one cannot write. This vast feeling of emptiness, like a choke hold.

*

I didn't think Ronnie was a decade older than me when we met. She still looked like a girl, in her thrift knee-length skirts and her porcelain skin and her high-pitched, whispery voice. At first I thought of her as cheerful—well, we were all supposed to act cheerful, up, smiley, in such environs. She still had a girlish figure, because she didn't eat, because we didn't eat then, we couldn't afford it, not really—we ate what they fed us if we worked in the food industry, usually on discount. If we paid for food, then we would have no money for coffee or vintage dresses or makeup, which we usually didn't anyway.

She would buy the most beautiful makeup—almost period pieces—pink puffs for powder, the most feminine little containers. I can still see her when she was going out at night, on a date, grooming herself elaborately. The way she'd hit the puff against her face.

I think someone like her had to remain a girl. She still worked "girl" jobs—bar girl, coffee girl, cigarette girl, etc. It keeps you, in a way, young. At least for a while.

Girls like Wanda and Ronnie were dependent on their looks to get by, even though they really didn't get by. Dependent on some man to take interest in them and buy them dinner, maybe help them out with groceries.

Wanda still had her looks. White trash but still white. White, blonde, blue-eyed. With the right clothes she could be the American girl.

*

In her review of *Wanda*, Pauline Kael calls the character Wanda a slut several times. Kael was fond of the word. In the same essay in *The New Yorker*, she also calls Elaine May's character in *Mikey and Nicky* a slut. I wonder how Barbara Loden registered the shocks when she read the review. Wanda is "an attractive girl but such a sad, ignorant slut that there's nowhere for her and the picture to go but down . . ." She also writes that Wanda is "too numb to be a competent hooker." I don't think Kael really got how Loden was showing her character being pulled slowly through life, drifting into situations. She has no money. She has no real place to stay. She must fuck these men to get by. She finds herself, the next day, squinty-eyed in a strange bed.

*

After the factory incident, Wanda is picked up at a bar by a balding salesman in a bad suit. When he buys her a beer, she holds her face in one hand, pours it, not even registering him. The next scene she's naked in bed, sleeping; he is dressing quickly, trying to leave. When she wakes up and sees him, she dresses hurriedly as well, pulling on her sad holey underwear, running out after him, her hair now a ponytail on top of her head. Wanda's hair is a recurring absurdity in the film. In the first scenes, her hair is wrapped up in a scarf in curlers. But then when we finally see it down, her hair is pin-straight and fine, and all she can manage is that ponytail. Mr. Dennis, the petty criminal she falls in with who has quixotic dreams of grand larceny, demands that she fix her hair. What would I do with it? she asks, in her way. A hat or something, he demands. When he gives her money, she buys a silly headband decorated with plastic daisies at Woolworth's.

The businessman tries to shake her off at an ice cream stand, speeding away as she's ordering. Handed the cone, she stares out at the highway. She sets off walking. She wanders into a department store, staring at the mannequins behind the glass wearing outfits she cannot afford.

Ronnie would window-shop at night, walking down Damen Avenue in Bucktown past the storefront boutiques after they had closed. Cheaper that way, she would say. Like Agnès Varda's pop-star blonde Cléo, played by

Corinne Marchand, in *Cléo from 5 to 7*, trying on hats. Except she cannot afford anything.

Wanda is more like the drifter played by Sandrine Bonnaire in Varda's later *Vagabond*, in the French *Sans toit ni loi* ("without roof or law"). Wanda wanders into a Mexican cinema, only to fall asleep and, upon waking up, find her wallet gone.

Then she walks, unknowingly, into the midst of a robbery. The man she will call Mr. Dennis throughout the film is behind the bar when she walks in, an unseen man tied up at his feet. Mr. Dennis is played as a twitchy loose cannon by Michael Higgins, who also plays the brother of the Elia Kazan stand-in in Kazan's autobiographical film *The Arrangement*, a send-up of his early relationship with Loden. She is bold for the first time in the film. She eats the potato chips in the bowl and asks for something to drink. She startles him. He clumsily pours her a glass of beer. "You want to know what happened to me? Someone stole all of my money," she tells him, unaware of the irony of her appeal. She asks him for a comb, which he, still startled, pulls out of his front pocket, nervously looking at the door. She pulls it through her bangs—such a clumsy, childlike gesture.

Later we will of course see them naked in bed. He freaks out at her when she touches him. "I don't like friendly people." He brusquely tells her to get up and get dressed and get hamburgers, with exacting directions. He's violent and abusive and impenetrable. He makes her pick the onions off of his hamburger. She does it because he tells her to.

She eats sloppily too—the potato chips, the spaghetti at the diner he later takes her to. He is impatient, paternalistic. "Wipe your mouth, will you?" She obeys.

I write in my notebook when I rewatch this scene: "THE GIRL IS A HOT MESS." I also write: "THIS ESSAY IS A HOT MESS."

The draft is chaos. The draft is a form of disaster.

*

For some reason it is excruciating forcing myself to rewatch *Wanda* for this essay, even though it is one of my favorite films. I procrastinated over watching it for days. Something to do with empathy.

I think I felt suffocated from intense waves of empathy while waiting tables at the Hollywood. I met more Wandas there too, women rather brutalized by life. My fellow waitresses supporting too many family members, the ones who got abortions and had to go to work the same day, the one who came to work with bruises because her boyfriend beat her up. The old ladies I'd work that afternoon shift with—one had terrible emphysema but still fiercely held on to her menthols; she once was hospitalized and still had to scramble to cover her shift. She was the mother of another waitress there who worked the lucrative early-bird shift, whose teenage daughter had been missing for some time—she showed me a photo of her staring from a poster, blonde like her, not as hard yet. Lost. The other waitress on that afternoon shift lived alone, would slowly shuffle home afterwards, with her liter of Pepsi and her plastic bag of videos from the Blockbuster that she'd watch at home. She was friends with the diabetic lady who would sit at the counter spooning up her hot chocolate.

*

The rest of the film leads up to the bank robbery Mr. Dennis plans that inevitably will fail. They embark on a strange road trip odyssey in a stolen car, including stopping at a fake catacombs/tourist trap for Mr. Dennis to visit his elderly father. Mr. Dennis has Wanda read out loud from the newspaper article about the bar robbery as he drives. She slowly picks at the text like a young child, then the slow realization. "Hey, what are you trying to get me into," she freaks out, pushes the newspaper at him. He has no patience for this display of willfulness.

"Get out—" He opens the door. Yet her flicker of resistance has gone out. We only see it once again, at the end, when she fights against a soldier on leave who is trying to rape her. "I didn't do anything," she pouts. She stays. She doesn't have anywhere else to go.

*

An incongruous moment of *Wanda* that I love: Mr. Dennis, in a gesture that can either be described as gross or touching, and maybe both (the beauty of this film is how many moments cut across these two concepts), lays his meaty, sweaty hand on Wanda's thigh while they are driving on the highway. He palms her thigh and she lets him. How Hollywood taut and tan that thigh is. A burst of autobiography. In reality Barbara Loden was the much younger wife to this much more famous man.

The orphaned misfit meeting the married director twenty-three years her senior while a dancing girl at the Copacabana nightclub in NYC. Like something out of that Marilyn Monroe film *Bus Stop*.

In the film, Mr. Dennis is the harsh director; Wanda is his actress. He instructs her not to wear makeup. To only wear dresses—throwing her newly purchased slacks out onto the highway as Wanda stares at them wistfully. He directs her for her role in the robbery, where they plan to hold a bank executive hostage in his house—she is in costume as a pregnant woman needing to make a phone call as she knocks on his door. Throughout she lets him. It is as if she has been looking for someone to tell her what to do.

*

On YouTube there is a video of Barbara Loden on *The Mike Douglas Show*, when Yoko Ono and John Lennon cohosted. She is promoting *Wanda*. She narrates, in her quiet, self-effacing way, that she met the famous couple at the Cannes Film Festival. Here she has long shiny gorgeous hair; she is wearing knee-high boots over white jeans and a brown flowy peasant top. (I keep on pausing and trying to figure out whether these are the same white jeans worn in *Wanda*.) She is a bit reserved, which she discusses with the famous couple, their mutual shyness.

One of the first things Mike Douglas asks, after noting positive attention to *Wanda*, the critic's prize it won at the Venice Film Festival: "Does your husband have anything to do, does he stick his toes in anywhere, when you're filmmaking?" She handles it politely. "We help each other." "How does he feel about you making your own films, Barbara?" "Well, umm, he was the one who made me do it. It never entered my mind to make a film. I had no ambition that way." The North Carolina accent comes out. She sounds, suddenly, so much like Wanda. She repeats: "He made me do it. He forced me."

Barbara Loden lived under her husband's shadow for years, until she broke out when she made *Wanda*. After that, she began to be more confident in her identity as a filmmaker.

Kazan was upset that she had abandoned her role as a housewife. He had actually begun divorce proceedings, until she found a lump in her breast. She was to die eight years later at the age of forty-eight.

He writes in his autobiography, "When I first met her, she had little choice but to depend on her sexual appeal. But after *Wanda* she no longer needed to be that way, no longer wore clothes that dramatised her lure, no longer came on as a frail, uncertain woman who depended on men who had the power . . . I realised I was losing her, but I was also losing interest in her struggle . . . She was careless about managing the house, let it fall apart, and I am an old-fashioned man." A mirroring of the court scene in *Wanda*, the grievances of Wanda's husband.

Later, he still claimed that he wrote the screenplay to *Wanda* himself.

*

The most intimate moment in the film is when Wanda and Mr. Dennis are sitting on the car in a field, eating and drinking beer. He puts his coat on her. He looks at her. He asks her why she doesn't dress herself up nicely. She tells him she doesn't have any money to get new clothes. "I don't have anything, never did have anything, never will have anything," she says quickly, lightly, eating delicately. "Stupid," he says to her. "I'm stupid," she says, shrugging. "You don't want anything, you won't have anything. You don't have anything, you're nothing, you may as well be dead," he lectures her. "Well, I guess I'm dead then," she says. He gets mad at her. She shrugs and doesn't make eye contact. In the next scene he's given her money to buy clothes.

This scene reminds me so much of Ronnie. The same lilting voice. Her being so immobilized at times by the uselessness of her fate. Learned helplessness. The going inwards.

In truth Ronnie and I were both depressives. And by that I mean we wanted to have contact with other people, but often found fatiguing the casual, accepted exchange. Social encounters both made us feel somehow unseen, and then drained, so we were more likely to go inwards. This made us revolt, in different ways.

That eternal question "What do you do?" We could not answer in any way that explained things properly. For what we did did not define us. Although we did not actually know what did define us. Ronnie especially would become enraged at that question. I witnessed this at the occasional social gatherings we went to together. She would often retort something snippy. "I am a professional Ronnie." That was her line. I was still so nice all the time then. I couldn't imagine how someone could be not nice. I was always so embarrassed, but also impressed, that she could transcend niceness. In some ways she reminded me of my prickly, secretive mother I loved so intensely. There was a connection there. One year my mother invited Ronnie home for Easter. I don't think Ronnie ever forgot that kindness. I can still see her across the room at my mother's wake, sitting alone on that island of an ottoman at the suburban funeral home, dabbing her eyes with tissues. She must have read about it in the newspaper. As I said, we'd been out of touch for some time.

I think in some ways I thought of my observations of Ronnie as a sort of film in which I could reconstruct my mother's mythical secretary days, her eating tomato sauce on crackers while being a struggling single mother to my half sister, living poor on Chicago's west side until my father saved her, setting her up in rather mundane lower-middle-class suburbia. She always said that when my father asked her to marry him he assured her she didn't have to work anymore. Although of course she worked—

scrubbing kitchen floors at 5 AM on her hands and knees. When courting her, he'd bring her heads of lettuce and sticks of salami.

I always thought that the only escape for Ronnie—and this is terrible—was marriage. She wanted to settle down, I think. To be taken care of. At that point in her life that was Ronnie's only option, or so it seemed to me then. She only went to that one year of community college. She didn't have money for more school. She didn't really understand how to use a computer, even though she once dragged home an ancient yellowing PC to try to get it to work, set it on her grandmother's Formica kitchen table. She was tired of temporary dead-end jobs. She didn't want to work like that any longer.

*

I don't know why people call them salad days. None of us ate salads then.

At the diner the waitresses had to prepare the salads. We were supposed to put on plastic gloves. We would be sitting around the corner of the counter, chain-smoking and playing go fish and looking at catalogues of china figurines that all the mom waitresses were crazy about. Then we'd have to prepare a little shitty iceberg salad, slathering on the ranch dressing.

*

Nobody—nothing. A cipher. The consummate actress shifting identities to please. "I used to be a lot like that," Loden told the *Los Angeles Times* in 1971, adding: "I had no identity of my own. I just became whatever I thought people wanted me to become."

*

There was that time Ronnie fell in love with the scholar of postmodern fiction who was much older than she was, who resembled something like a well-oiled mole—I didn't get the appeal, except that he was an adult who owned his own place. I think perhaps it was about the idea of him more than anything—what he represented, how he could potentially change her fate. How loving him could be a career in a way. While he was away for the summer, she shut herself up in her bedroom and read all of the big massive tomes of the postmodern novelist whom he specialized in. As if she could get closer to him through the object of his obsession.

And of course he broke her heart, cruelly, suddenly. It didn't mean as much to him. How could it? He didn't want anything permanent.

Mr. Dennis, for all of his abuse, does love Wanda. He loves her because he sees her. In that moment, them sitting on the car, he sees her.

The film, in its way, is a strange, fucked-up love story. They are the opposite of the glamorous Bonnie and Clyde. Loden maintained in interviews that she thought of her film as an anti–*Bonnie and Clyde*. She also made clear that although the films came out at around the same time, she wrote the screenplay years before.

Faye Dunaway was Barbara Loden's understudy in *After the Fall*, which Elia Kazan directed, where Loden played the Marilyn Monroe apparition.

Dunaway then later played the Barbara Loden muse figure in the film version of *The Arrangement* with Kirk Douglas as the antihero—even though Loden was promised the part. After all it was about her. Or Kazan's version of her.

In Kazan's autobiographical novel, *The Arrangement*, the mistress character, Gwen, is a spitfire apparition whose role is to provoke his character, to shake him out of his complacency, his numb bourgeois existence as an advertising exec. In their life, Loden was the one who pushed him to start writing screenplays.

In *The Arrangement*, the Barbara Loden figure is a one-dimensional sexpot. "But Gwen had no closed doors, no forbidden rooms."

After a small part in his film *Wild River*, Kazan cast Barbara Loden a year later as the flapper Ginny Stamper in *Splendor in the Grass*, who pushes her brother, Warren Beatty, to come out from under the thumb of their domineering father. In that mint-green cloche hat shooting daggers at the judging church congregation. "I hate it here! I'm a freak in this town." In blonde curls playing her ukulele, such fury and glee against the disapproving father. In Clara Bow red hair with that spit curl, dancing around in her underwear and thigh-highs, flap-flapping around, powdering her armpits, humming *she's the talk of the town*.

A manic performance as opposed to the minimalism of Wanda. In *Wanda* Loden gives a performance stripped of anything. We only get her amazing face, both open and closed, her bruised looks, her mumbling speech. Her staring out at the highway, like into outer space. Her collaborators on *Wanda* portrayed her as "sensitive," as "insecure," and yet Kazan in his autobiography depicted her as a "bitch," as "white trash."

*

Sometimes Ronnie and I would share horror stories of our breakdowns. She told me she was once so depressed she shit the bed. I feel a betrayal writing this. But that's what she told me.

I never saw Ronnie cry. But I saw Ronnie vomit because she was so heartbroken and depressed over the rejection by the scholar.

No one mourned like Ronnie. When that man broke her heart, she shut herself inside her little room, sleeping on emptied cereal bowls, spoons, fashion magazines. She was immoveable. I recorded this site of absolute devastation somewhere inside of me and resurrected it for the depression scene in *Green Girl*, where my Ruth, a blonde, slippery, impenetrable girl, recovers from something like a broken heart through the relief found in catatonia.

Maybe that's why Lol Stein is so fixated on the past— going back to her traumatic scene of rejection. The last time she felt that eruption of intense emotion, having her heart destroyed.

*

In my published novel the breakdown scene is much shorter than the version I first wrote. Originally I had

Ruth stay inside and sleep all day for at least thirty pages. Pages upon pages on her dirty mattress on the floor, shuffling back and forth from the fridge, watching screens until she was bleary-eyed. Everyone who read it told me to cut it down. All that depression—who wants to read it? They didn't understand the grand spectacle, the funereal ritual she needed to undergo. And also I wanted to somehow convey the boredom and banality of being depressed.

*

At first during the time he's away John and I talk on the phone or Skype a couple times a day. He wants to see my face, see the puppy. Eventually we Gchat once a day. I find it more of a fluid mode of communication. I need to tell someone how lonely I am. How in the morning I'm busy, taking care of the dog, making food for myself. But how I spend afternoons curled up on Genet's dog bed.

*

At the end, everything awash in miserabilism, alone again, no partner in crime, Wanda becomes paralyzed. She sits at a bar as the television announcer narrates the event, the bank robbery a terrible failure, Mr. Dennis shot dead. She allows a soldier to pour drinks into her. She only wakes up when he drives her to the desert and forces himself on her. Her high-pitched scream. She escapes into a forest, breaks down into tears. At the end, she wanders into another bar, finds herself in a booth, people talking at her, giving her a cigarette, a drink, a hot dog—she accepts them all wordlessly, numbed out again. All dirty blonde ponytail, dazed and grasping her drink amidst the blur of the bar crowd.

In her review of *Wanda*, Pauline Kael expresses horror at the character's catatonia, her lack of empowerment. She writes: "It's such an extremely drab and limited piece of realism that it makes Zola seem like musical comedy. Wanda is a passive, bedraggled dummy. We've all known dumb girls, and we've all known unhappy girls; the same girls are not often, I think, both dumb and unhappy."

*

The Appalachian woman in *Airless Spaces* reminds me of Wanda. Debra Daugherty "an obviously once beautiful chick who now looked like a wasted Appalachian from a Dorothea Lange photograph of the thirties. In other words 'white trash.'" All day lying on the couch in the main area complaining. Later living in a "trashed" Section 8 apartment on Avenue D in NYC. Her family gave her Clinique makeup for Christmas (my mother and those yellow bottles of moisturizer, the free giveaways).

*

The depressed, ambitious Esther Greenwood in Sylvia Plath's *The Bell Jar* fantasizes of changing into a girl she calls Elly Higginbottom. This imagined alter ego is a simple girl, who wants nothing more than to be married to some sailor and have lots of children.

Of course the story of Wanda is a reminder that even muted girls can be terribly sad. The violence that they internalize.

I wonder in a way if Ronnie is my Elly Higginbottom, my alter ego. Like Wanda was for Barbara Loden. Some sort of twinning. Perhaps the objects of our obsession, our characters we fictionalize, can be a way to try to figure out something of ourselves, of our pasts, how our presents could have been different somehow.

*

"What do you do all day?" My new therapist has that discomfiting way of looking directly at me. I have started regular therapy, for the first time in many years. The insomnia has returned, the night sweats, the tingling through my veins, a bomb inside of my body with hair triggers.

It might also have had something to do with the fleas. They came on as soon as John returned. A plague of them. Something to do with the abnormally warm winter. I think we both went deranged. We would see one little black speck crawling around Genet's deflated ball sack, and the day would suddenly be overthrown. All day cleaning and vacuuming. We began to wake up in the middle of the night and throw our sheets off to see if we could see any black stains on the white. The raised red map of persistent bites around my knee and left thigh, where Genet curls into me while we're sleeping. I was itching constantly. I think I had some sort of allergic reaction. I began to think bugs were crawling on me all the time.

I chose my therapist because she went to Harvard and worked in the DBT ward at McLean. She is a tiny woman, about my age, with a halo of frizzy hair, who wears airy pastel skirts. She looks a bit like David Mamet's wife, that actress who plays neurotic roles. She has an old-fashioned name that suits her. I don't think she particularly likes me. No charm offensive works on her.

Although I liked the idea that she worked with wrist cutters and tortured girls, I want to remind her I am not one of them. I am not mute and stubborn. I am, instead, hyperverbal, eloquent, discussing psychological theories and concepts. Still she corners me on my tics of self-deprecation. When I tell her that I struggle with feelings of inferiority, with convictions as to my own stupidity.

Writer's block. How boring. I am supposed to be working on an essay, this essay in fact, but something stalls me. I cannot enter into it. I am unsure what is the use of all of this first person anymore.

*

In *Airless Spaces* the narrator remembers being medicated and sleeping all day after the hospital. So much about the tyranny of the day within the hospital. Every minute controlled and accounted for so one doesn't go off schedule.

*

What do you do all day? I am looking for anything to do to distract myself. I wouldn't be a good fictional character in a short story because I surround myself with other screens. I watch anything. I find myself on YouTube looking at videos of David Letterman interviewing starlets. All of their shiny, hard legs—Emma Watson, Claire Danes, Katie Holmes. Katie Holmes has this summer announced her separation from Tom Cruise. I wonder how many others have gone to these videos recently, to attempt to trace out any meaningful emotion or interiority amidst the banal cheerisms and the typical flirtation, the fingers through unbearably glossy hair. Something about having to wear a mask over the loneliness—or perhaps not even allowing the monologue to rise up at all.

The fantasy narrative is that she is a suppressed wife who suddenly is free from a Svengali husband. That she has experienced an awakening.

After *Wanda*, Barbara Loden planned on directing a film adaptation of Kate Chopin's *The Awakening*, a turn-of-the-century novel about a woman who comes into her own as an artist, and decides she wants a life outside of being mother and wife.

Edna Pontellier, like Wanda, is a passive character. Like Wanda, but more like Lily Bart in *The House of Mirth*. At the beginning she is viewed as an object, a commodity, by her husband, who likes to collect expensive things. She allows herself to be collected. She never questions the way society is supposed to go. Simone de Beauvoir writing of the Wife in *The Second Sex*: "The temptation to forgo liberty and become a thing."

Those silk dresses Ronnie would keep in a box in the closet, and that she would take out, from time to time, to stroke lovingly. Remnants from the past. Gifts from a former lover. Like Sasha's fur coat in *Good Morning, Midnight*.

I find myself watching a video of Katie Holmes going out for ice cream in New York with her daughter. I feel totally creepy doing this. "Katie and Suri Spotted Smiling."

In *The Awakening*, Edna is the expensive wife whose days are segmented. All the oppressive rules and rituals that sink her soul, make her unexplainably depressed. She finds a temporary freedom when her days open up, in the summer. In the city, in New Orleans, she becomes a flâneuse, walking, circling, wondering. Coming into consciousness.

*

I'd like to imagine Loden playing Edna in her version of *The Awakening*. It is the part she was meant to play. I'd like to see her in a different register. A different layer of autobiography. The existentially trapped wife who becomes the tentative artist. It makes sense that Loden would move on from the abject poor wife to the wealthy one.

I wonder how Barbara Loden would have played Edna. I only know her as the femme fatale or the frozen Lavinia, her hands and tongue cut off, who allowed brutality to happen to her. The woman who murders or the woman who is murdered. I would like to see her play someone closer to who she was. The artist woman. The smiling woman who realizes her society is a trap. Who doesn't wish to be surveilled any longer. Who wants to attain sovereignty.

In *The Awakening*, Edna Pontellier begins to spend all day painting, even begins to find some financial independence as a painter. With *Wanda* too, Barbara Loden became an artist.

Edna giving herself up in ecstasy to Mademoiselle Reisz's piano—the music stirring something in her soul that makes her see herself anew. Apparently Ronnie studied to be a classical musician, but then gave up. I don't know why. She wouldn't talk about it. You couldn't get her to. She'd just close up. She'd shrug her shoulders and go inwards. She didn't even have her instrument anymore. She had hocked it. I mean, I understood that. At some point I too had pawned all of my expensive things, although all I really had were expensive junky things, the gold jewelry given to me for my confirmation.

One of her occasional jobs was as a telemarketer for the Chicago Symphony and sometimes she would get free tickets. She was always trying to get me to go with her. I never did. But I can imagine her sitting there silently, yet offering herself up to the music. She knew how to enjoy things more than I did. I always admired that about her.

*

In therapy we discuss my reluctance for publicity, my anxieties and nerves over reviews of this new book I have coming out that's about my obsession with the lives of famous literary wives, how personal reviews can seem. How I google myself constantly. There is no sense, from her, that any of this fear and loathing might come out of the culture, the sense of badness and dumbness and failure I carry around with me as a woman, as a woman writer.

I feel, when she tells me I judge myself, that she is judging me for judging myself, and this makes me feel angsty.

A writer I just met offers to ask her Jungian analyst if she'll Skype in with me for occasional sessions, just to get me through the fall. "You'd be better off having a Goodreads reviewer as a therapist," she writes me over email, about this woman I drive for a half hour to go see once a week in Durham.

Even though I feel myself resistant, even though she doesn't take my insurance, I keep on returning to her. I feel, somehow, that I want to please her.

*

I can't imagine what Barbara Loden must have thought when she read Pauline Kael's acidic dismissal in *The New Yorker*. Although there are small praises (Loden's gift for "character"), the overall pronouncement is that this is a small, muted film, too small, too muted, with two unlikeable characters. In other words, a failure. Not worthy. Did she take it personally? Did she go in passively, inwards, like a shot in the arm? Like Wanda reacts passively, as if expected, to Mr. Dennis's critical pronouncements.

Kate Chopin was also ostracized when she wrote *The Awakening*; her beautiful book was dismissed for decades. Reviewers of *The Awakening* were not only morally outraged about this narrative of a woman who wants something outside of marriage, but also dismissive that her "torments" were worthy of literature.

*

What do you do all day? I'm always curious about others' quotidians. More than anything I want to know what people do when they are alone.

Although I'm enthralled to others' quotidians, I don't know how to write it, let alone how to live it.

In *The Bell Jar* Esther feels trapped in her mother's house in the suburbs one long blank summer. She cannot figure out how to survive her days.

How to structure your days: the question of the depressive as well as the writer. How does one write when there's no way to break up time?

My therapist encourages me to follow a practice of mindfulness. As I'm beginning to understand it, mindfulness is an attempt to live and exist in the actual world, even when it's slow or boring or uncomfortable or painful.

The example she gives is being mindful when going to the bathroom. I hate when people say "going to the bathroom." She says be aware of everything, of opening the door, of sitting down, of turning the faucet on, of carefully washing one's hands. When I walk into the little house that holds her practice in Durham, I often see a patient coming out of the bathroom, walking slowly, slowly, down the hall.

*

Ronnie somehow managed to exist through her days. Even when unemployed. I think she was a model of solitude for me. She knew how to soothe herself. She would take long, luxurious baths with these little French soaps she bought. Even when she had no money she would go to the dollar store and buy little things that amused her.

She was religious about the rituals of coffee. She would wake up in the morning, her hair curtaining off her face, and prepare her French press, and pour it into her grandmother's china cups, and she would drink it all day, even when the milk became sluggish. She would wade through the *New York Times* all day every Sunday. She subsisted mostly on coffee and popcorn. She would make a big bowl of popcorn and would nibble at it all day. The stale chewiness of cold popcorn. Sometimes she would make a pot of chicken soup, putting in a whole bone-less chicken that she dragged home from the Jewel off of Ashland, and we would eat that all week.

*

My mindfulness exercises are often of the domestic variety. I attempt to thoughtfully, meditatively prepare food and fold laundry, all the real-life activities I have been shirking. As I slowly and inexpertly chop onions, I think about this. Even though I am trying so hard, to be free of distractions and noise, of a cycle of anxiety and negative thinking, I am not sure I want to be a completely balanced, enlightened person. And what is the difference between this concept of mindfulness and the domestic monotony of Jeanne Dielman, Chantal Akerman's Belgian housewife? I guess it's all in perspective.

I saw online an image of a page of Sylvia Plath's journal, where she reflected on reading Virginia Woolf's diary. And how gratified she was to learn that Virginia Woolf also became the good housewife when she was dreading reviews of her book. I read this and I feel some sort of doubling, link, with both of them.

*

I have begun swimming. It helps me work off excess nerves. Like an edge has been taken off. I am calmer, more open afterwards. I swim at the local community pool. I try to avoid the snarls of hair on the benches, like filthy lures.

There is hardly a moment of exercise when I am not keeping time, anticipating when I can get out of the pool, when my twenty minutes is up. In the filter at the shallow side I always stop to regard some object washed up. A soaked-through cigarette butt. A wad of chewing gum. A filthy Band-Aid. A spider.

The other day a woman in a bright pink bathing suit, wearing what looked under the bright turquoise water to be black socks, bobbed gently up and down as she walked in a lane in the open swim area. As I allowed myself a break, panting short, jerky inhales, I watched her. I realized she was lifting white Styrofoam weights at her sides as she bobbed gently up and down. Up and down. Forcing legs through the water. As if in a trance.

Sometimes, rarely, I forget the choke of the chlorine in the bright blue pool, forget the bored guard watching me from the deep end, forget the hair clogged and my environment entirely. The chill of the deep. The warmth of the shallow.

When swimming I sometimes think through this essay. The body essays. It attempts.

It is the experience of swimming that reminds Edna Pontellier in *The Awakening* of the freedom of her childhood, running through the grasses of Kentucky. It is open to interpretation, the ending, whether she drowns or she becomes one with the sea, like a goddess shuffling off all the restrictions of society, mortality, morality, maternity, wifedom. I guess it depends how you look at it.

*

Elia Kazan writes in his autobiography that when Barbara Loden died, she died in fury and excruciating pain. The cancer had spread to her liver. Her last words—"Shit! Shit! Shit!"

I wonder if Barbara Loden thought of her film career as a failure. Whether she measured herself against the success of her husband, his films that are now seen as classics. The screenplays she could not get funded. She died a decade after *Wanda* came out. The film only played in one theater in New York.

"There's so much I didn't achieve, but I tried to be independent and to create my own way," she wrote. "Otherwise, I would have become like Wanda, all my life just floating around."

I'm drawn—always—to failures. To the aborted project. Edna Pontellier was supposed to be a bohemian painter, and move to Paris, and then she got scared. She was not strong enough to fly away from prejudice. The hag pianist Mademoiselle Reisz tapping her shoulder blades, her fragile wings. Wanda got lost on the way to the bank robbery. And lost again in the ambiguous ending scene— never really found. Yes, Barbara Loden was, in a way, in terms of concepts of career and the canon, a failure.

And yet the work survives. This singular work.

*

A few years ago I was watching a video online of a sit-in downtown in a health insurance office, protesting for single-payer healthcare. Of the protesters being dragged away by police I recognized Ronnie, kicking and screaming. I searched for her online for a few hours and made out that she was now involved in several activist groups. I also observed, rather cynically, that she was also dating someone involved in one of the groups.

I contacted her on Facebook to say hello. She said hello, cordially, back. But then I realized she blocked me.

I mean, I understand. Sometimes one desires to sever off the past. But did she have a political awakening, a coming-to-consciousness? Or did she change, at least initially, for someone new in her life? Impossible to know, I suppose. I hope that it's the former—that she found her voice.

I hope, wherever she is, that she is happy. No, happiness sounds so trite. I hope that she's fulfilled. I wonder if she still makes popcorn all the time.

ACKNOWLEDGMENTS

Grateful acknowledgment to the editors of the journals and collections in which the following stories and essays appeared, sometimes in slightly different form:

BOMB: "Susan Sontag," "The Fourth Annual Jean Seberg International Film Festival," "Introductions to B. Ingrid Olson"; *Anne Collier* (MCA Monographs): "Fragments of a Lost Object: Meditations on the Photographs of Anne Collier"; *Apogee*: "Sleepless Nights"; *Fireflies #5: Agnès Varda/Angela Schanelec*: "Gleaning"; *Frequencies* (Two Dollar Radio): "One Can Be Dumb and Unhappy at Exactly the Same Time: An Essay on Failure, the Depressed Muse, and Barbara Loden's *Wanda*"; *Icon* (Feminist Press): "New York City in 2013: On Kathy Acker"; *Paris Review*: "Blanchot in a Supermarket Parking Lot,"

"Second Dog," "Plagiarism," "Diane Arbus Visits Marilyn Minter in Gainsville, Florida."

Thank you to the Sarah Charlesworth estate and Paula Cooper Gallery for permission for the wonderful Sarah Charlesworth collage for the cover. Thank you to Mónica de la Torre at *BOMB* especially. Gratitude to Emily Nemens and Hasan Altaf at *The Paris Review* for publishing four pieces in their spring issue. Thank you to B. Ingrid Olson, for asking me to write a series of texts inspired by her work, which were typeset and photographed by the artist and included in her show at the Albright-Knox Art Gallery in Buffalo, New York. Thank you to Sarah McCarry and Jenny Zhang, for giving me the opportunity to write "Sleepless Nights" on the occasion of the Guillotine launch of *Hags*. Thanks to Amy Scholder for asking me to write about Kathy Acker, and Eric and Eliza at Two Dollar Radio for asking me to write about anything, at any length. Profound thanks to Mel Flashman. Thanks to everyone at Harper Perennial, especially Sarah Haugen, Caitlin Hurst, and Amy Baker. Thanks to Mary Beth Constant for her witty and succinct copyedits. Thanks to Brian Evenson, Amber Sparks, Wayne Koestenbaum, and Jen George. Gratitude and love to Sofia S., Danielle, Suzanne, Steph, Clutch, Amina, Hedi, Cal, and Bhanu. Love to Leo, whose face I watch with such joy. And as always gratitude to John.

ABOUT THE AUTHOR

Kate Zambreno is also the author of two novels and three books of nonfiction. She lives in New York and teaches writing at Columbia University and Sarah Lawrence College.